TIPS FOR IMPROVING YOUR HEALTH

RECOMMENDATIONS FROM THE PROPHET MUHAMMAD A.S.

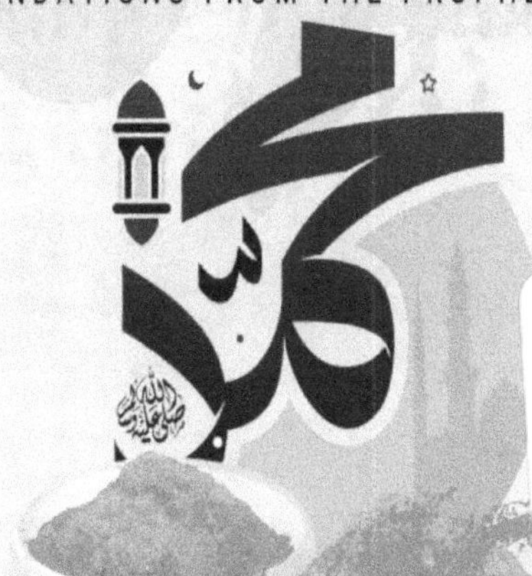

TIMURLENK CHEKOVIKJ

Tips for imroving your health

Recommendations from the Prophet Muhammad ﷺ

Timurlenk Chekovikj

2020

To my blessed mother

Table of Contents

Introduction

Medicine is a science that thoroughly deals with physical and human health, prevention, and treatment. It dates as much as the human race itself and has always had a special place in society with its related disciplines. Because of this, Islam from the very beginning had a prominent role with the intention of building a healthy community. Anyone who will study the life of God's messengers, and especially the life of the Last Messenger of God, Muhammad ﷺ[1], will find that they gave a special place and importance to medicine. Their whole life is full of wisdom and advice on how to improve one's morals and health.

As narrated by Imam Ahmed[2] : *"I came to the Prophet, peace be upon him, and found him with his companions. They were calm and serene as if there were birds over their heads. I greeted them and sat down. Then some Bedouins came from various places. They asked him: 'O Allah's Messenger! Should we seek medical treatment for our illnesses?' He replied: 'Yes, you should seek medical treatment, because Allah, the Exalted, has let no disease exist without providing for its cure, except for one ailment, namely, old age'."* [3]
With their guidance and counseling, God's messengers lead people to a healthy way of life and, by practical examples, encouraged them to practice and learn many important sciences.[4] It fostered the spirit of firm intention in patients and the sick, while doctors led them to seek the "*right cure*" for every disease. The Messenger of God ﷺ said: *"Every disease has a cure and when an appropriate cure is applied to the disease, it will pass with God's help."*[5] It is also said in another narration that: *"Allah*[6]

did not send down any disease but that He also sent down the cure."[7]

At the point when the patient feels that there is a solution for each malady, his heart is moved by the spirit of expectation, the warmth of despondency vanishes, the door of hopefulness opens and the soul recovers, along these lines restoring its intrinsic mental and characteristic educational encounters.

At the point when natural frameworks are fortified they become a positive power that will beat the illness. A similar rule applies to the specialist who, when he understands that the patient's ailment has a cure, will attempt to ingrain extra expectation in the patient. Consequently the health problem of the body and that of the heart is comparative.

For each sickness of the heart, Allah has made a intravenous injection - that is its opposite. At the point when somebody whose heart is wiped out will perceive the ailment and mend it with its resistance and he will recuperate it by God's arrangement. For instance, eagerness is treated with modesty, tension with a positive mindset, a condition of dread is treated with boldness, melancholy, and withdrawal are treated with tranquility and receptiveness in correspondence thus like.

In this book, you will get to know a short reference list of medicine utilized by the Prophet Muhammad ﷺ and which he suggested to use. We will present you the part of cleanliness, smart dieting, fasting, just as the unsafe outcomes of certain items and propensities.

The advantages of optimism, prayer, internal struggle, as well as the sociological aspect, are presented at the end of the book. All of this contribution is only a small part of the research we have presented to our readers, and it originates from Islamic civilization.

These researches and recommendations nowadays can significantly help in the treatment, therapeutic, and other uses and treatments that can be part of the modern research and development of medicine. While reading, please think about the organs in your body - you have developed from a single drop of seed to a certain extent, and then the development halts. Each organ has its own precisely determined size and function and all together in magnificent harmony make up the human body. If individual organs continued to grow in moderation, what would the human body look like? Imagine the human whose hands would be dragged on the ground! Or the man with an apple-sized head! Or...! So do you know who "programmed" those small drops to "grow" and "develop" to certain limits and who gave all the organs that make up man to grow?

The intention was not to make an ordinary book but to be acquainted with the advantages and a call for research in the topics presented.

The development of Islamic medicine throughout history

Adhering to the viable directions of the Last Messenger of God ﷺ, Muslims in the early time of the new age in an exceptionally brief timeframe progressed medication by turning into its pioneers. Examining clinical science, they outperformed Greek, Persian, and other clinical sciences, and for quite a long time their work was indispensable for all educational institutions. As ahead of schedule as the eighth and ninth hundreds of years, Arab medicine thrived. Schools were set up to interpret Arabic into Persian, Indian, and Greek to make them accessible. Because of the Arabs, all works by Galen and Hippocrates were saved. Simultaneously, the Arab researchers distributed their works that plundered Europe for quite a long time to come.

Around then, Baghdad alone had around 600 clinics, while Cordoba in Spain had more than 500 clinics. State-subsidized, these medical clinics additionally had a logical instructive job, and because they were state-financed, they had their libraries, clinical schools, and centers, just as different therapy units.

However, the first mobile Muslim military hospital was that of Rafid al-Eslami to which the Prophet Muhammad ﷺ ordered to perform his duties towards the wounded and sick in a mobile tent. Islam encouraged women to heal the sick, which was its purpose in the first battles of Islam, healing the wounded and bandaging their wounds. Among them was Keiba bin Saad Eslami, who wrapped the sick and wounded in her tent.[8]

Pharmacy and botany,[9] during the Islamic renaissance are studied not only as a separate science but also included the areas within medicine. Almost all Islamic scholars wrote about these areas to put these two scientific fields in the service of medicine. The pharmacy was a science that greatly attracted Muslims. Gustav Lubon says: "The science of pharmacy can be attributed to Muslims without any hesitation, and we can say that this science is a real Arab-Islamic invention."[10] One of the most significant contributions of Muslims to this science is the introduction of a system of remedy inspection and surveillance.[11]

At the time of the Ma'mun reign(786-833), there was a ban on the arbitrary practice of pharmacy, and this area of medicine was placed under state supervision. At this point, ruler Ma'mun was accused of many scams by self-proclaimed pharmacists who claimed to have cures for all diseases. Because the sick did not know the medicine, the pharmacists were able to proscribe the sick any medicine.

So, Ma'mun ordered a pharmacist confidentiality test. Afterward, Mu'atesim (795-841) ordered the issue of a license to operate in the field of pharmacy, the one for who is determined that is reliable and has enough knowledge. Thus the pharmacy entered the general system of inspection[12] which further spread to various parts of Europe during the reign of Frederick II (1210 - 1250).

Max Meyer Hoff, a german orientalist, said: "Pharmacy studies written at this time cannot be counted. These studies were about natural remedies that were not (artificially) composed of components, and the most famous author of those studies was Ibn al-Baytar.[13] He is one of the greatest scientists to have written about plants in Arabic. "[14] Ibn al-Baytar in his work *Compendium on Remedies* showed how and in what way we can get the medicine by processing plants, animals, and minerals. He fully embraced the achievements of the ancient Greeks in the fields of pharmacy, biology, and mineralogy.[18]He had in mind the *Anatomy* of Galen and the *Flora* of Pedanius Dioscorides. In al-Tazkirat, Dawud al-Antaki paid special attention to the season of harvesting the plants, the way of storage, and the zonal distribution of the plant world, and Ibn an-Nafis in the treatment of infectious diseases relied more on regulating the patient's diet than on its use. In the height, because it was boycotted by the Arab pharmacists. However, despite this, Ibn an-Nefis have devoted some parts of his great work to the pharmacy.

In the preparation of plants and the synthesis (the composition of medicines), Muslim pharmacists used new methods, and some of those methods are still used today.[15] In the field of pharmacy, Muslim doctors have made many significant discoveries. They were the first to describe coffee beans as a remedy for the heart, and the fruit of coffee (ground coffee) as a remedy for inflamed tonsils, diarrhea, and inflamed wounds; indicated that the comfort tree improves the work of the heart; adding lemon juice, orange or cinnamon and cloves reduces the strength of some remedys; discovered some antidotes that made up dozens or hundreds of remedys; improved the synthesis of opium and mercury, used herbs and opium and other anesthetics.[16]

It is quite obvious that Muslim scientists have played a major role in laying the foundations of pharmacy, and in its development and expansion. They wrote special works on pharmacy and so it became a real science.[17] Ibn Sina devoted some parts of his great work *Canon to medicine* and pharmacy. In his paper, he described many medicinal plants and minerals that produced various remedys. Similarly, Al-Biruni, Ibn al-Haytham, Sabit ibn Qura, Ar-Razi, and other Arab scholars have written great and very important works in this field.

Al-Idrisi described many species of medicinal and other plants in his *Botany*.[19] Muhammad ibn Yusuf al-Hawarizmi and Abdurrahman ad-Dawni were great pharmacists. First of them, in his book *Miftahu-n-Ulum* resonates with the study of various diseases writing about simple and complex medicines prepared from plants and various minerals such as mastic, hyacinth, ginger, Mirta, Citrus, phosphorus plant's extracts, milk, and various resins. The second, in the work *Nuzechtu-n-nufusi ve-l-efkari fi marifeti-n-nebati* besides the description of the other plant and mineral origin and the possibility of their application in medicine, spoke about the composition and preparation of the poisons, essential oils, and fats.

Al-Kurtubi is among the famous Arab pharmacists. In the work *Interpretation of Names,* he explained how and in what method we can get the medicine supplement by processing plant, animal, and mineral raw materials. Of medicinal plants whose products are used as raw materials in the manufacturing of the remedies he mentioned: Nigella Sativa (black seed), mustard and minerals dark blue vitriol, borax, copper sulfate, vermilion, and from animals he mentioned the crow and some others.

Muhammad ibn Zekeriya ar Razi (865-925) wrote a book about children's diseases and many consider him the father of pediatrics and his capital work *Jaundice* belongs to one of the first of this kind to diagnose this disease. Scientist Ar Razi was the first to use mercury in dairy products, and this research was applied to monkeys. He also advocated for the medical use of chemical compounds.

Sabur Ibn Sahl (869) was the first doctor who encouraged the development of pharmaceuticals, describing many remedies and medicines against diseases.

Abu al-Qasim al-Zahrawi (936-1013) begin the preparation of medicines by sublimation and distillation. His *Liber servitoris* is of particular interest, providing the reader with a prescription and explanation of how to prepare the "simplest" medicines, which are later supplemented by the commonly used medicines.

Al-Biruni (973-1050) wrote one of the most valuable Islamic works on pharmacology, entitled *Kitab al-Saydalah* (The Book of Remedies), which provided detailed information on the properties of remedies, he stressed the role of pharmaceuticals, as well as the functions and duties of pharmacists.

Abu Ali al-Husayn ibn Sina (Lat. *Avicena*; 980-1037) was the first to codify the medical science of his time and world-famous encyclopedic work: The *Law of Medicine*. This masterpiece is precious and has been translated into Latin several times during that time. It has made an enormous contribution to modern medicine, and medical students in Europe have been educated on it for centuries. For many European scientists, Ibn Sina is one of the greatest medical scientists of all time. Ibn Sina also described no less than 700 preparations of medicines, their properties, mode of action, and their instructions. He has devoted an entire volume of simple remedies in the canon of medicine. [20]

Another Arab explorer Ibn Isaac was Huneyn (lat. *Joanitus*; 809-873) was known for his book of ophthalmology under the name " *10 discussions on the eye* ".

Abdulmalek Ibn Zuhr (Lat. *Avenzoar;* 1091-1162) from Cordoba was the first to discuss bone diseases, osteoporosis, scurvy, and others.

Ibn Rushd (Latin *Averroes* 1126-1198) wrote the well-known work entitled "The *Comprehensiveness of Medical Science* ".

However, the works of *al-Maridini* from Baghdad and Cairo and *Ibn al-Wafid* (1008-1074), which were printed in Latin more than fifty times, also had a great influence. *Al-Muwaffaq, who was* living in the 10th century, wrote The *Establishment of the True Properties of Medicines*, where he described, among other things, arsenolite oxide and introduced us to silicic acid. He made a clear distinction between sodium carbonate and potassium carbonate and drew attention to the natural toxic compounds of copper, especially copper sulfate and lead compounds. He also describes the distillation of seawater for drinking.[21]

Ali Ibn Nafis (1210-1288) wrote the *Explanation of the Commentary on Ibn Sinan's Code,* in which he advanced his knowledge of pulmonary circulation three centuries before the Portuguese Servetus, to whom the work is attributed, did the same.

In the 13th century lived the medical historian Ibn Abu Usayb who in his work *Biographical Data of Physicians* collected over 400 biographies of famous Arab and Greek physicians. In addition to the above, many other names have decorated Arab-Islamic history. They made a great contribution to the evolution of world medicine and modern knowledge.

Many facts in the field of medicine in the last decade only confirm the Divine nature of Islam. God's faith offers us a healthy life, forbids everything harmful such as alcohol, drugs, prostitution, and empowers a healthy life that consists of moderate eating and drinking, cleanliness of the body, maintaining good habits.

Despite the great advancement of technology, the billions of dollars invested in health, more and more people are getting sick and dying from various diseases. According to world statistics, 10% of people die of old age, 20% from various wars and accidents, while 70% die from various diseases. It is indicative that lately, a growing number of diseases that were not known before and which are becoming a major challenge for the fast-growing world population are spreading. Especially, the danger of viruses is considerably great.

In this book, you will learn about the ways of healing in Islam, guided by the motto *better to prevent than to cure*. We will first get aware of the medicine that the Prophet Muhammad ﷺ did teach us, on the principles of healthy living, the great importance of hygiene, diet, sleep, physical activity, etc. The short encyclopedia of some of the medicines is to be aware which natural medicines and herbs are recommended by the Prophet ﷺ. They contributed to the construction of better human moral codes and norms of behavior, as well as protection from infectious diseases, general hygiene, and human health in contrast to the European cities which were sinking into famine, poverty, infectious diseases, and ignorance. Muslims have used prophetic advice successfully for the last 14 centuries and have helped the development of medicine and pharmacy.

At present, modern medicine and natural remedies can not be imagined without this important chapter of history which is yet to reveal its rich possibilities and knowledge of the advantage and healing of the recommendations and norms set by the Prophet of Islam.

Islam and health

Islam as a perfect way of life pays special attention to the protection of human life. At the same time, it reminds us that health is one of the many blessings of God that Allah has bestowed on many, but at the same time, it is a temptation for man to act towards that grace. Muhammad ﷺ reminded us of the value of health with the words: *"Pray to Allah for health! "No one has been given anything more precious after akin (firm belief) than health or cleansing from sins."*[22]

Muhammad ﷺ himself prayed for health in this world and the hereafter, invoking prayers in the morning and evening: *"O Allah, I pray for the health in this world and the Hereafter, O Allah, I ask for forgiveness and health in my faith and my life. "*[23]

They asked the Messenger of God ﷺ: *"Allah's Messenger, teach me something that I will ask from Almighty Allah." He said, "Ask for health.".* [26] Health, after Islam, is the greatest blessing to the human race because a man without health can not fully and delightfully perform all obligations to his Lord, so he should be thankful to Allah.

However, people throughout history, and even today, in which everything is seen through the prism of matter and interest, have considered that material wealth is something most valuable, the most precious that man can possess, forgetting the importance of health. But when a person temporarily loses his health, he becomes ready to give up everything he has, just to be cured. The problem is that most people are not aware of what they have until they lose it. An Arabic proverb about this attitude reads: " *Health is the crown on the head of healthy people, it is seen only by those who are sick.* "

Health is a precious reward of God that most people misuse and exercise in violating Allah's commands and acting on prohibitions. In this regard, Muhammad ﷺ in one of his prudent sayings said:

"Many people are deceived by two benefits: health and leisure." [27] That is, they do not know and appreciate their value. The benefit of health is one of the five most important things for a person whose importance was especially emphasized by the Messenger of Allah. He advised his ummah[28] to improve for Judgment Day. The Prophet ﷺ said:

"Use five things before you are hit by five others: life before death, health before illness, young before old age, wealth before poverty, and free time before busyness." [29]

One should be thankful to Allah and not forget Him, even though Allah (SWT)[30] may deprive him of some benefits. A person may have one leg amputated, but one should ask what is the condition of those who have lost two legs. A person may be blind in one eye, but what about those who are blind and can not see at all? Such thinking can strengthen a person psychologically and give him the strength to more resolutely prolong his life and wait for the reward of temptation.[31]

Purity and hygiene in Islam

Muhammad ﷺ said, " *Purity is one half of the faith* ."[32] This has been confirmed by science, as hygiene does prevent numerous infectious and other diseases. Therefore, the believer through prayer[33] which is obligatory together with ablution[34], must constantly maintain hygiene several times a day. This includes bathing, which is mandatory at least once a week, especially on Friday (Friday). Bathing is obligatory after the intimate relationship with a partner, after a woman's menstruation, and it is also desirable after the unpleasant smell of the body from sweat and work.

Nail trimming and hair removal are emphasized in the famous tradition of the five innate qualities that were a tradition and practice of former Prophets. The Messenger of Allah ﷺ said: *"There are five innate natural properties: circumcision, washing the pubic hair, cutting nails, removing underarm hair, and trimming the mustache."*[35]

The human body needs to eat and drink to stay strong and productive. Food is an essential element for maintaining a healthy body. That is why we distinguish how Islam commands the believer to eat permissible and delightful things. The Almighty says:

"O you who have believed, eat from the good things which We have provided for you, and be grateful to Allah if it is [indeed] Him that you worship." (Qur'an; Baqara, 172)

From that point of view, Islam forbids certain things to its followers, exclusively because of their harmfulness. A

Muslim is strictly forbidden from consuming alcohol, and a reasonable person is aware of its harmful consequences.

So basically everything harmful is forbidden to man, which is a great indicator of the perfection of Islam and its immeasurable concern for human health. Imagine the benefits of banning prostitution, which today is a major cause of many incurable diseases worldwide such as AIDS, Syphilis, Gonorrhea, Tripper, etc.

As we have already mentioned, Islam has prescribed treatment and seeking medicine in case of illness. Muhammad ﷺ ordered a treatment through fasting, so he said: *"Fasting is a shield and protection (from disease)."* [36] He also said, *" Indeed, you have duties to perform towards your body."*[37]

Allah in the Qur'an also indicates a special kind of medicine, and that is honey. Muhammad ﷺ noted: *"Hold on to two medicines: the Qur'an and honey."*[38]

The golden rule is that *prevention is worth more than a chiliad of medicines.* Today, with the development of medicine, with the development of the technique and the examinations that have been performed, the recommendations of Muhammad ﷺ are direct evidence of the supernatural content of his words, as well as the practice he did not instruct.

Immune system - "army" of the Almighty

Each day there is a war going on in our inner parts of our body, and we do not even become aware of it. On one side are the viruses and bacteria that want to enter our body and bring it under control, and on the other side are the immune cells that protect our body from these enemies.

Enemies act offensively to find a way to the desired area, which they aspire to enter as soon as the first useful opportunity is presented to them. However, strong, organized, and disciplined soldiers (immune cells) in the attacked areas will not allow their enemies to succeed in their intentions so easily. Primary, "soldiers" destroy and neutralize "enemy soldiers" (phagocytes) upon arrival on the battlefield. But sometimes the battle is "harder" than these soldiers could handle. In such circumstances, other soldiers (macrophages) are called to "fight". Their participation causes alarm in the attacked area and other soldiers (auxiliary T-cells) are called in the battle.

These soldiers know the local population well. They quickly distinguish their army from the enemy. Immediately activate soldiers who have the role of producing weapons (B-cells). These soldiers have exceptional capabilities. Although they have never seen the enemy before, they can develop weapons that will disable them. Also, they carry weapons that they create so quickly that they can use immediately. During this journey, they succeed in the difficult task of not causing any harm to the allies. Later, the attacking crews arrive (deadly T-cells). These deadly T-cells fire poisonous material, which they carry with them, to the most sensitive enemy points. In the case of victory, another group of soldiers comes to the battlefield (suppressing T-cells) and sends all the soldiers back to their camp. The soldiers who arrive last at the battlefield (memory cells) record all the information about the enemy, so that they can use in case of a similar invasion in the future.

The wonderful army we are talking about is the immune system in the human body. All of the above are performed by microscopic cells invisible to the naked eye. How many people are aware that they have such an organized, disciplined, and perfect army in their bodies?

How many of them are aware that they are surrounded by microbes that if not prevented can cause serious illness or even death. Indeed, there are many dangerous microbes in the air we breathe, in the water we drink, the food we consume and the surfaces we touch, although man is unaware of all these events, the cells in his body make tremendous efforts to save him from the disease which could even cause death. The ability of all immune cells to distinguish enemy cells from domestic cells in the body is very interesting, the ability of B-cells to prepare weapons to neutralize an enemy they have never seen before, their ability to create enough weapons they need to use without adverse effect on any cell of the body. These are just some of the striking features of this system.

It is very difficult for a person to survive if he does not have an immune system, or if it is malfunctioning because he would be exposed to all the microbes and viruses that are found in the outside world. Nowadays, such people can only live in specially designed rooms without any contact or anything in the area. Therefore, a person without an immune system can't survive in a normal environment. Is it not ridiculous for the unbelievers to claim that all this happened by some natural coincidence, and Allah says in the Qur'an for those who have a reason:

"We will show them Our signs in the Universe and within themselves until it becomes clear to them that it is the truth. But is it not sufficient concerning your Lord that He is, over all things, a Witness?"[39]

The perception of pain is part of the body's defenses. Pain warns us of the danger of damaging the integrity of tissues by triggering an adequate defensive reaction.

Nociception is the neurophysiological term for the specific activity of the nerve pathways that conduct pain. These pathways mainly carry information - pain, but which the brain does not have to interpret as such.

All pain receptors are free nerve endings that are widespread throughout the body. There are mechanical, thermal, and chemical pain receptors. They are found in the skin[40] both on the inner surfaces as well as on the outer covering of the bones and the articular surfaces. The deep inner surfaces are poorly supplied with pain receptors and they propagate a feeling of chronic, severe pain if tissue damage occurs. Therefore, a detailed description of the patient is of great importance for the assessment and successful treatment of pain.

The doctor should know that pain must be unconditionally relieved, because it damages primarily the nervous system, but also damages the cardiovascular, respiratory, gastrointestinal, endocrine, immunological, and other systems in the body. Suffering from pain is not only uncomfortable but also harmful.

A short encyclopedia of the Prophet's medicines

The Prophet treated with three types of medicines: natural, divine, and combined medicines. Although Islam has not excluded modern pharmacy, natural remedies that the Prophet ﷺ used are described and explained.

Aloe vera

Aloe is an herb that is known long ago as the elixir of long life. The healing properties of the essential oils have long been known in ancient times. It was used by the ancient Egyptians, and in tropical Africa, it was used as an antidote to the stings of poison arrows. The ancient Greeks and Romans used it to heal wounds. It has also been used for its beneficial effects on the digestive system.

Uthman ibn Affan, radiyallahu anhu, narrates a hadith in which it is stated that a man complained to the Prophet ﷺ for pain in the eyes during the pilgrimage, after which the Prophet ﷺ told him to cover them with aloe.[41] Aloe vera gel has also been used to treat ulcers and infections of the mouth and eyes. If aloe is mixed with other drugs, it removes their negative effects on humans. It is used to treat swollen eyelids, liver, jaundice, and to treat abdominal blisters. Aloe vera stem is also useful against cough and vomiting. It also strengthens the heart and senses. Aloe Vera is a plant that is found in the tropics and subtropics and belongs to the family of vines, not cactus, as it seems and as most of us call it. The plant is stemless, with saber-toothed leaves about 75-120 cm long, light green that is serrated at the ends and forms a rose in the middle with a stalk on top of which is a yellow or reddish flower.

Contains over 240 nutrients and healing ingredients that include: amino acids needed for tissue growth and development, enzymes, minerals (calcium, iron, magnesium, manganese, sodium, copper, zinc, potassium, aluminum), vitamins (A, B1, B2, B3, B6, B12, C, E), as well as folic acid, choline, inositol, niacin.

With the number of useful vitamins and minerals, aloe has an immunostimulatory effect on the human body. Aloe contains the following healing properties: strengthens the body's resistance, detoxifying - cleanses the body of toxic substances and various chemical substances, antioxidant, antiviral, antibacterial, analgesic, antidiabetic. Helps with many infectious, rheumatic, lung, blood, nerve, benign and malignant diseases. Aloe leaf juice is a great cleanser for the intestines and is very useful in case of constipation. Also, aloe is ideal at home as first aid for burns and wounds, for fungal infections, and helps with inflammation of the veins.

FDA (Food and Drug Administration) has approved its use in the treatment of eye diseases, sports medicine, dentistry, and internal use. We should know that the American FDA is one of the strictest food and drug control institutes in the world.

Antimony (Usmud)

Antimony strengthens the optical fibers and protects the eyes. The Prophet said: *"The best medicine for the eyes is antimony. It strengthens the eyesight and enlarges the lashes. "*[42]

He also said: *"The best medicine is antimony. It protects the healthy but not the sore eye. "*[43]

Tirmidhi also conveys a legend stating that Prophet had a special container in which he kept the antimony. He applied antimony ointment to his eyes three times each night. A similar hadith is narrated from Enes r.a. through Abdul Latif that the Prophet Muhammad ﷺ said: *"Antimony increases the growth of eyelashes, beautifies them, and that is why our hearts love it. "*[44]

According to the latest research, it cures *Schistosomiasis* (a parasitic disease) as well as various skin diseases, and

Chinese scientists claim that antimony is a cure for leukemia. In large quantities the antimony is poisonous.

Banana

".. and among the banana trees (Talh) with fruits strung .." [45]

Ibn Abbas states that this tree is similar to the reproductive structure whose fruits are sweeter than honey and describes it as arranged and has no spines, and bears more fruit. Talh is the name used by the people of Yemen at that time. The banana has a sweet taste and a soft, creamy texture. It is quite enough that this fruit is part of our daily diet. Given that it is available to us and consumed throughout the year, it is important to know its basic advantages.

Banana is a great source of potassium that helps maintain normal blood pressure. Besides, potassium is good for the bones, kidneys, and bones. Bananas are also rich in probiotics that are great for the digestive system. They are rich in vitamin B6, vitamin C, magnesium, riboflavin, and iron.

They are practical for consumer goods and are a great snack. They are healthy enough that they are even part of the daily diet of babies. One banana has only 100 calories. You can also combine them with cereals, protein shakes, yogurt, or other fruits in a fruit salad.

Behar Palm Tree

Palm trees are tropical plants, most often on a coast, ie. beach. Perennial plants, whose fruits (like dates) are very tasty.

Allah (SWA) says:

"And tall palm-trees, with shoots of fruit-stalks piled one over another,"[46]

The Almighty says: ***"In them will be fruits and palm trees and pomegranates."***[47]

Transmitted by Aliya r.a. that he said: *"Respect the palm tree because it was created from the same land from which Adem a.s. "*

The Prophet once asked the Companions[48] which tree most closely resembles the Muslim. After several wrong answers, the Prophet ﷺ said: *"No, it's the Palm tree".* [49] Palm trees are one of the most famous and cultivated plant families. From them are obtained various products and food items, and they are appreciated because of their value as ornamental plants in the exterior.

Basil

Basil is warm. Its aroma strengthens the heart. Water sprayed with basil makes us sleepy. Bukhari narrates the following hadith:

"If someone offers you basil, do not refuse it, because it is simple to use and has a pleasant smell."

Basil in the form of tea is used to treat inflammation and diseases of the urinary tract. This soothing spice relieve coughs and hoarseness and helps treat cold sores. Basil oil is considered to be an excellent remedy against acne. Basil has been used as a spice and vegetable for centuries. If used as a spice, it stimulates the appetite and has a beneficial effect on the digestion and balance of the intestinal flora. Also, it can help diabetics, as it lowers blood sugar levels.

In the form of tea, it is most often used in the treatment of inflammation (stomach, intestines) and diseases of the urinary tract (kidneys, bladder).

Basil oil also has a beneficial effect on the nervous system, soothes tension, migraines, improves memory, and removes mental fatigue.

Basil dressings improve wound healing. Fresh basil leaves are known as a home remedy for insect bites.

Grapes (Vitis)

"With it, He causes to grow for you the crops, the olives, the date-palms, the grapes, and every kind of fruit. Verily!.."[50]

The vineyard is a blessed plant - a plant that is mentioned in almost all the holy books, the Torah, the Psalms, the Gospel, and the Noble Qur'an, and was cultivated 6,000 years ago. The origin of the vineyard is from Central Asia (near the Caspian Sea) and even today you can find grapes in its first form. Its original remains have been found in Bronze Age artifacts as well as in the cemeteries of ancient Egypt. Grapes are also mentioned in the time of the Prophet Noah. Today the largest growers of grapes are Italy, France, and the United States. This fruit plant is mentioned in the Qur'an 11 times, and it grows and is produced in good climatic conditions.

Unfortunately, we have not implemented it properly, and not as much as it should in our religious life. Grapes in small quantities can be planted and grown in our gardens, as well as in large pots, in our homes. Fresh grapes are low in calories because they contain 80% water. Grapes are low in sodium and low in fatty acids and cholesterol.

Due to dehydration, raisins contain more calories and are a good source of iron for the anemic (people with poor blood). About 25% of grapes are composed of sugar. Grape sugar penetrates the blood vessels very quickly, so it is very effective for physical fatigue even after treatment for the anemic disease. Due to the high concentration of iron, grapes stimulate blood regeneration and are used as a natural remedy for the liver, kidneys, and digestive system. Grapes stimulate the functioning of the kidneys and due to the regulation of the excretion of excess fluid from the body, it reduces high blood pressure.

 Drinking grape juice is recommended for those who suffer from stomach ulcers, gastritis, inflammation of the shoulders, rheumatism, damage to the liver, and spleen, as well as some types of poisoning. Grapes strengthen the heart muscle, help treat bronchitis and cough, neuralgia, and insomnia. It cleanses the blood and improves skin tone. Dry spark grapes help respiratory diseases, prevents the intensity of coughing, kidney pains, those of the urethra, and is considered an effective tool in improving memory. It is narrated from Ibn Abbas that the Prophet ﷺ said:

"Eat the raisins but throw away the seeds because in them is the disease and the rest is medicine."

It is one of the richest sources of boron, a mineral that has been shown to reduce bone loss in menopausal women. The mineral was discovered in 1808, and research has shown that it is a very important element for healthy bones. The richest sources of pine are soy, dried figs, raisins, peanuts, hazelnuts, and walnuts. Grapes today have become the focus of several scientific studies. In 1996, scientists discovered a substance in it called *resveratrol,* which showed excellent anti-cancer quality. This substance has a great effect against cancer in three stages, and because of that, it is an extremely effective means of natural chemotherapy.

It is worth noting that these healing compositions of grapes are not found only in summer. Of course, the sincere believer has this in mind and it is quite clear to him because: *"And from the fruits of the date palm and the vineyard, you take a drink and pleasant food. In that, indeed, is a sign for the people who understand. "*[51]

Quince

Talha r.a. reports that the Prophet gave him a quince and told him: " *Eat it because it calms the heart."*[52]

Ibn Majah also narrates the following hadith: *"Eat quinces because they calm the heart, and Allah (SWT) did not send a messenger without giving him to eat, because it gave him strength like at least 40 people."*[53]

There is also another hadith about quinces which says: *"Let your pregnant women eat quinces because they make the heart softer and better."*[54] A "softer heart" means that quince injects tenderness and kindness into the heart. Quince also reduces blood flow during the menstrual cycle in women. Eating quince after a meal relaxes the stomach, but if we eat too much then it causes stomach cramps. Quince syrup is good for coughs and sore throats. Quince cream refreshes the veins and strengthens the stomach.

Ginger

Ginger is mentioned in the Qur'an:
"And they will drink glasses of ginger in it."[55] ,

"And there they will be given a cup whose mixture is of Zanjabil (ginger). A fountain there, called Salsabil.".[57]

The ginger tea mentioned in this Qur'an is a recipe for a healthy lung and a healthy body. It is a recipe from heavens. narrates Said Abu hadith that the Byzantine emperor sent him a jar full of ginger as a gift to the Prophet ﷺ which he divided and ate with the Companions.

Ginger did not arrive in Europe until the 15th century after the Crusades, and it was widely used as a medicine. Ginger is warm, sweet, and tastes like lemon. Ginger also expand blood vessels. Ginger increases appetite stimulates the sex drive and stops gas. Ginger syrup soothes the stomach and helps the immune system.

Ginger is also good for the elderly, especially those suffering from severe inflammatory diseases. It is one of the most famous plants in the world. The underground ginger stem is used as a spice in the diet and is also useful in alternative medicine. Ginger is a perennial cabbage plant that grows mostly in the tropics part of the Earth. The plant grows and reaches a height of up to 1 meter, and its roots are as thick as a finger, 20 cm long and are very aromatic. The flowers are white, yellow, or pink depending on the species. More than 2,000 years ago, ginger was mentioned in medical books as one of the ingredients in many oriental medical recipes.

Ginger may be consumed fresh, antecedently exposed to steam or dried, also grounded into a powder. contemporary ginger was used as a remedy for innate reflex, cough, and flatulence (increased gas within the organic process system), biological process ginger powder was used as a remedy for abdominal pain, shortness of breath, nausea, lumbago, and looseness of the bowels. Africans use ginger root as a decent aphrodisiac, whereas Papua ladies use ginger root as a contraceptive. In India, contemporary ginger tea is used as a cough reliever and as a remedy for occlusion.

Ginger has many medicative properties and is especially used as a decent medication. Researchers have tried that ginger is best than pharmaceutical medicine against nausea, that prevents the sensation that produces an individual vomit.

Ginger doesn't cause sleepiness as a result of it acts on the abdomen, not the brain. This ability of the gum brewage was utilized by sailors on long voyages, by mastication acid ginger, overcaming nausea caused by the large ocean waves. To stop nausea, it absolutely was necessary to consume solely 0.5 a teaspoon of ground ginger in juice, tea, or food.

Researchers in Denmark have found that ginger is effective against blood clots as a result of it prevents the synthesis of a substance known as thromboxane that signals blood cells to clump, that is that the beginning in coagulum formation. Researchers at Cornell University have found that ginger thins the blood and breaks down blood clots with the assistance of a substance known as gingerol, that encompasses a structure very like acetylsalicylic acid, that is additionally called a decent medication.

Researchers in India have found that ginger drastically reduces the high level of cholesterol in the blood caused by the uncontrolled use of saturated fats in the diet. In Japan, ginger has been found to reduce pain (analgesic), prevent vomiting, reduce the excessive production of gastric juice, reduce high blood pressure, and stimulate the heart. Ginger has also been shown to block unnecessary mutations in human genes that lead to cancer.

Cereals

Allah says: *The proof is the dead earth: We give it life, and from it sprout the grain which they eat;* [58]

We send down blessed water from the sky, and with its help, We cause gardens and grain to sprout, [59]

The Rahman chapter also highlights the benefits of grain:
and grain with weeds and leaves on the stems,
So which of the favors of your Lord would you deny?[60]

Cereals were a major source of food in history. Proteins and carbohydrates in cereals make the base of the food pyramid, and many of them are forgotten and unnecessarily thrown from the daily menu. Buckwheat originates from Asia and appears from Tibet, China, and Japan from where it has spread throughout Europe. Buckwheat lately becomes second in popularity, unlike other cereals that were needlessly neglected. The Latin name *Panicum miliaceum is a* name for millet, extremely rich in iron and magnesium, and also contains calcium, phosphorus, zinc, iodine, sulfur and vitamin B complex. Like other cereals, this one helps regulate the work of the intestinal microflora that has a positive effect on the work of the nervous system. So, it improves the condition of patients with arthritis. It is prepared as a side dish, especially as a porridge in which you can add fruit of your choice or as part of pudding or similar desserts; it can be fried, mashed, salad and alike. Millet flour is especially suitable for preparing eggless cakes. The origin of these cereals is from Arabia and Egypt; widespread use is especially in Asia, China-Japan, and India. Barley is also widely applied in kitchens around the world, and fed the ancient civilizations of Egypt, Greece, Rome, Israel, and Tibet. The Prophet Muhammad ﷺ did not indulge in regular consumption of cereals but mainly ate barley and barley bread. It is reported by Aisha, r.a.: *"If someone was exhausted, the Prophet ﷺ would order barley soup to be prepared and sipped, and then He would say, 'It strengthens the heart of the sorrowful and moves the heart of the sick as water removes the filthiness from your faces.' "*[61] Barley is easily digestible and therefore the Prophet ﷺ recommended the use of barley- *talbina* soup, which is used for all stomach aches. Barley is prepared with fruit as porridge, like crumbs, in soups, it is made into malt that replaces sugar. It is rich in minerals such as potassium, sulfur, sodium, iron, manganese, phosphorus, iodine, vitamin b complex.

Apple cider vinegar

Muhammad ﷺ said: *"The best of the spices is vinegar.*[62] Also transmitted through Xhabir b. Abdullah that the Messenger ﷺ said: ".. *bring it to the target because it is a good food supplement (spice)."*

Why Muhammad ﷺ recommended vinegar? We know that the Prophet ﷺ spoke nothing of his own mind. His actions are an example for us and today and the food he used are part of scientific recognition of the uniqueness of it in medical and other purposes.

Apple cider vinegar is a cure for various diseases. Elderly people know it as the biggest enemy of obesity, but apple cider vinegar has an antibacterial action, kills bacteria, fungi, and other microorganisms, and helps fight viruses.

Apple cider vinegar is rich in minerals, vitamins, and other substances. Contains vitamin C, vitamins E, A, P, B1, B2, and B6. Among the most important minerals and vitamins in apple cider vinegar is pectin, which helps maintain a healthy diet. Consuming apple cider vinegar for weight loss is a practice that is thought to have started in ancient Egypt. Vinegar helps cleanse the liver, speeds up metabolism, burns calories, and reduces appetite.

In recent years, industrial production of apple cider vinegar has been observed, but it is indisputable that domestically produced apple cider vinegar has an advantage over industrial production. Apple cider vinegar is first and foremost a food that has healing properties and gives a special quality to the daily diet. It can be used as a spice in salads and as a side dish or simply put in a glass of lukewarm water and honey and drunk. It can also be placed on a cotton swab to clean some parts of the body.

 Apple cider vinegar is an excellent antiseptic and is often used to cleanse the skin. In such cases it is used diluted with water, depending on the purpose and the age. Apple cider vinegar is best taken one tablespoon at a time, with two teaspoons mixed with a glass of lukewarm water. Potassium in apple cider vinegar, along with other ingredients, dilutes the blood and helps control blood pressure.

The fiber in apple cider vinegar helps absorb cholesterol and remove it from the body as waste material. Dietary fiber in apple cider vinegar also helps control blood glucose. Arthritis usually causes the storage of metabolic toxic waste in tissues. Apple cider vinegar helps speed up metabolism and flush out toxins. Minerals, such as magnesium, calcium, manganese, silicon, and iron develop bone mass and make bones stronger.

Apple vinegar is useful for treating infections such as candida which causes an imbalance of alkaline and acidity in the body. A solution of apple cider vinegar and lukewarm water immediately relieves the symptoms. Apple vinegar treats block our airways colds and flu. The discomfort can be significantly reduced if apple cider vinegar and black pepper are applied to the chest. For a sore throat, gargle with a solution of apple cider vinegar and water. Apple cider vinegar can prevent food poisoning. Relieves constipation and stops diarrhea.

Pomegranate

The princely pomegranate, ar-Rumm in Arabic, is mentioned in the Qur'an as one of the many delicious rewards awaiting in Paradise. Its numerous uses in cooking and medicine, as well as its beautiful structure, make the fruit a wonder for Muslims who believe that each pomegranate seed is a sign of the Sustainer.
 Pomegranates are mentioned three times in the Qur'an as one of the fruits that will be found in paradise:
"In both of them are fruit and palm trees and pomegranates. So which of the favors of your Lord would you deny?" (Qur'an, 55:68-69)

As a reminder of God's sustenance on earth,

"And He, it is Who produces gardens (of the vine), trellised and untrellised, and palms and seed-produce of which the fruits are of various sorts, and olives and pomegranates, like and unlike; eat of its fruit when it bears fruit.."(Qur'an, 6:141)

And as a sign of his artistry,

"And it is He who sends down rain from the sky, and We produce thereby the growth of all things. We produce from it greenery from which We produce grains arranged in layers. And from the palm trees – of its emerging fruit are clusters hanging low. And [We produce] gardens of grapevines and olives and pomegranates, similar yet varied. Look at [each of] its fruit when it yields and [at] it's ripening. Indeed in that are signs for a people who believe." (Qur'an, 6:99)

The frequent mentions of this fruit owe to its gem-like beauty, a glistening core of seeds compacted in a layer resembling a honeycomb. Equally astounding are the colors of both the fruit and flowers which are an attestation to the Qur'anic verse:

"And whatsoever He has created for you on the earth of varying colors [and qualities from vegetation and fruits] and from animals. Verily! This is a sign for people who remember." (Qur'an, 16:13)

In the hadiths about the pomegranate, it is narrated by Enes bin Malik (r.a.) through the Prophet said: *"There is no pomegranate that does not have one of the pomegranates in Paradise in it. [64] Whenever Abbas r.a. passed by, he would eat a pomegranate seed. When people asked him why he did that, he replied: "I believe that there is not a single pomegranate and no seed in it that does not comes from the pomegranate of heaven, so maybe that is the pomegranate i ate."[65]*
Prophet said: *"The pomegranate and its bark strengthen the digestion (stomach). [66]*
Pomegranate (*Punica granatum*) is a shrub with low growth of deciduous trees that grow up to 5 meters in height. The origin is from Persia. It is mostly cultivated in Turkey, Tunisia, Spain, Iraq, China, California, Russia. In our country it succeeds mostly in the warmer parts of the country, Valandovo, Gevgelija, Dojran. Fertile and loose soil, protected from winds, suits her best. Maturation, depending on the variety is in the first decade of October to the third decade of October, the harvest is 2-3 times. The flower is bright red, very attractive, and blooms in several stages.
The fruits are 5-12 cm in diameter with a rounded hexagonal shape in which there are about 600 watery seeds that are red to purple. Pomegranates are rich in natural

nutrients and healing substances. In the diet, pomegranate is most often consumed as fresh juice, jelly, cold and hot sauces, thick syrup that is sweetened and is good as an addition to cocktails, to taste in cakes. Pomegranates look like red blood cells and have a wide range of light vitality. Pomegranate juice contains a large number of antioxidants, which protect the body from free radicals found in the blood. It is rich in vitamins A, C, E, B5, potassium, folic acid, and iron. [67] A glass of pomegranate juice reduces the risk of cardiovascular disease. It is one of the few plants that contain estrogen-like substances. Seed phytoestrogens can reduce menopausal and postmenopausal symptoms, including heatwaves.

Pomegranate also helps reduce the symptoms associated with aging. Studies have shown that it works to prevent the earliest chemical reactions that can lead to cancer. The plant hormones found in pomegranate reduce the risk of prostate cancer. However, there are a small number of studies that have examined the role of pomegranate juice in preventing the spread of prostate cancer, so further research is needed to determine with certainty whether it does have some benefit in cancer patients.

One study showed that pomegranate can reduce the amount of PSA in the blood. To improve PSA values, it is necessary to drink 250 ml of juice daily for several months.

Kana (Alkanna tinctorial)

Henna or Kana is cold and dry, although some say it contains heat. Used to treat blisters on the mouth and swelling. Heal and burns. It is also used as a hair dye and is good for treating nail infections. If someone has smallpox and rubs measles on their body, it will not damage it. Umm Seleme said: ***"The Prophet used to put henna on every*** *wound."*[68] Flower of Kana also considered useful for headaches caused by the blazing sun. The flowers should be left in acid and then applied to the forehead. Relief is easily achieved with this medicine quickly.

The book titled "History" from Bukhari states that a man complained to the Prophet ﷺ headache, and he l replied that it is the best hot bath of henna. While to the man who complained of pain in his legs he said: *"Smear them with henna."* [69] A hadith is also narrated from Abu Dawud in which he says that there is no plant more pleasing to Allah than Kana (Henna). Indeed, the cure for cuts is everything that removes excess moisture and stimulates tissue regeneration, and that is exactly the characteristics of henna. Removes excess fluid that slows down tissue regeneration. And when we put a henna flower on a woolen garment, it will give a nice smell and the moths will not attack it. Some claim that if we soak the henna leaves in water and then drain them and drink that water for 20 days, it will be possible to cure leprosy in its early stages. If the patient is not cured after eating and drinking this drink, then there is no hope for him.

Cucumber

The Prophet Muhammad ﷺ used to eat ripe dates with cucumbers.[70]

Such a procedure leads to the relief of stomach upsets and stomach acids. Whether you use cucumber in the salad or as a face mask, it is certainly useful. Due to a large amount of water, this type of vegetable is great, especially for weight loss. Cucumber consists of 95 % water. One who drinks a little water on hot days can make up for the lack of fluid in the body by eating cucumber, says Professor Hademar Bankhofer. In that 5% of cucumber, which does not contain water, there are many useful ingredients: magnesium, which is good against stress, potassium for the nerves, copper, which acts preventively against rheumatic pains and bitter ingredients that nourish the liver.

The most important enzyme in cucumber is erepsin, which facilitates the processing of proteins. Cucumber has few calories - in 100 grams it has 14 calories. Besides, it has a diuretic effect, ie it stimulates the expulsion of fluids and saturates quickly. It is eaten with the whole skin (only if it is organically grown) which contains ingredients that improve digestion. This vegetable is especially useful in the fight against aging. When you put cucumber on the face it absorbs water from it.

Watermelon

The Prophet often ate dates with watermelon and would say: *"This warms the body (the date) and this cools it (the watermelon)."*[71]
Interpreters explaining this hadith point out that by mixing the cold and warm effects of the two plants, the body is balanced and the energy is evenly distributed.
When we talk about this fruit it is important to say that no other fruit is as associated with summer like watermelon. In our country, watermelon is usually seen as a delicious sweet drink, but in reality, it is an energy bomb and a great natural remedy for many diseases. Watermelons are very rich in potassium, an element that helps regulate blood pressure, heart rate and can prevent heart attacks. Scientists believe that a diet rich in potassium prevents the

appearance of kidney stones and loss of bone strength in the elderly. Rich in fiber and completely free of cholesterol and fat, watermelon is an ideal food for those who want to lose weight.

Vitamin A, an antioxidant that is important for the eyes, is present in large quantities in watermelon, as well as vitamin C which helps to strengthen immunity, wounds to heal faster and easier, prevents cell damage, and protects teeth. Watermelon is also a source of vitamin B6, which helps with brain function and assists in the conversion of proteins into energy.

Until now, tomatoes were thought to be the richest in lycopene, but recent research shows that this is not true at all - no other fresh fruit or vegetable has been found to have as high levels of lycopene as watermelon. For those who do not know, lycopene is a super-powerful antioxidant that helps fight heart disease, cancer, and is especially effective in preventing prostate cancer and colon cancer. Watermelon contains large amounts of amino acids, citrulline, and arginine, which help the circulation and are crucial for the health of the heart and blood vessels.

When eating watermelon we should not limit ourselves to the red part - the seeds are very rich in magnesium and protein, and are highly recommended for those who follow a diet.

Fig

The Almighty swears by the great oath and mentions the fig tree: ***"I swear by the fig tree, the olive tree, and Mount Sinai."***[72]

It is narrated from the famous hadith of Abu Zerr that Abu Darda once offered the Messenger of Allah ﷺ *with a plate of fresh figs, so he turned and called everyone else to eat, saying: "Eat!, and he ate, and said:" If I had to say of some fruit that it was brought from Paradise, I would say this about this fruit because fruit in paradise has no seeds. It removes hemorrhoids and is good for bone pain! "*

Figs are very tasty and healthy fruit. The whole fig can be eaten from the outer shell to the sweet, red, fleshy middle part with small seeds.

Figs are fruits that are equally tasty and healthy, fresh, or dried. The value of the fig tree has been known for a long time, so throughout the history of mankind, the fig tree has been cultivated and consumed regularly. Figs fall into the category of oldest cultivated fruits. In the Mediterranean, it came from India via Turkey.

Figs with their nutritional composition and medicinal properties rise above many types of fruit. Figs are a better source of fiber than most fruits. About 28% of fig fibers are soluble. This type of fiber helps control blood sugar levels and lowers cholesterol levels, binding it to the intestines.

Studies show that consuming fruits rich in soluble fiber reduces energy intake, retains satiety instead of consuming foods with higher energy value. This means that fiber can help you lose weight.

Insoluble fiber from figs has a beneficial effect on colon health. They regulate digestion and allow normal bowel movements. Some estimates show that about 70% of cancer cases are related to poor nutrition. Most dietary theories have linked high fat intake and low fiber intake to colon cancer.

They act as antioxidants, blocking cancer-causing genes, and slowing the growth of cancer tissue. In addition to the usual polyphenols, figs also contain benzaldehyde and coumarin, which have been used successfully in cancer therapy. Fresh figs have a calming effect on airway inflammation.

The fig tree is a fruit that contains 80% water, sugar, and itself provides much energy that stimulates the brain, concentration, and memory. Natural fig sugars stimulate the brain. Given this, we can safely conclude that the fig is a favorite fruit of the brain. In natural folk medicine, it is known that ground figs are good for cleansing the skin, and also help treat acne on the skin. The leaves of the fig regulate insulin levels, so diabetics are advised to regularly use the tea leaves of fig.

Truffle (Tartuffe -Tuber)

The Prophet Muhammad ﷺ *said: "Tartuffe (tuber) is manna (honeydew)* [73] *and its juice is an eye medicine. "*[74]

The origin of the word truffle comes from the Latin *tuber*, which means lump, and growth. *Tuber* changed to *tufer*, hence the French name *Truffe*, the Spanish *Trufa*, the German *Trüffel,* and the Italian *Tartufo*. In world culinary readings you can find it as a diamond in cooking. You can also find in them many recipes called truffles, or truffles in one way or another, but it is rarely cooked with real truffles. Specialties often have this name because they look like them or are in some way related to truffles, or some synthesized substances have been used to replace truffles. You will recognize the dish in which real truffles are used, first at the enormously high price, and then by the unique smell.

Why so much fame about this food supplement?! Simple, it is rare, growth is in a specific way, and it is very expensive. Moreover, it added to the price because truffle can not be cultivated, although in the past there have been many attempts for wide cultivation.[75] Why this is so, there is still no concrete research and therefore truffles remain on the same level as real diamonds and pearls.

Truffles are sought after with specially trained dogs for this purpose. Some peculiarities of truffles according to current scientific knowledge

• Improves the work of all organs.

• Increases mental and physical activity.

• Increases the body's resistance to infections, ie has an antiseptic effect. Especially eye infections, conjunctivitis, etc., which is a confirmation of the words of the Prophet ﷺ.

• It is hygroscopic and binds, ie it removes excess water from the body and lowers blood pressure.

• It works against sneezing and colds as well as against dry cough.

• Cleanses the blood of toxins and is important in anemia.

• Increases the absorption of drugs and cleanses the body of harmful residues.

• Has aphrodisiac power.

• Helps to stop urination in children.

• Reduces pain tunic inflammation of the joints.

• Lack of enzymes - invertase and amylase, truffle prevents esophageal problems.

• Has a calming effect on the nervous system.

• Significant therapeutic drug for heart disorders due to the presence of acetylcholine.

• Truffle improves potency and libido. The decreased hormonal picture is especially pronounced in the period of menopause in women and andropause in men.

It is still a resounding name in the world of food, but also the world of the rich. They are found in most of Macedonia, especially in the southern Povardarie region. In Macedonia[76] the black truffle is found in Mariovo, Stogovo and Kumanovo, growing individually or in groups, under the soil, with young roots under woody plants, in humus on limestone substrates, under trees or shrubs, in deciduous and mixed forests with beech, cherry, ash, elm, as well as oak, pine, hazelnut, and spruce and up to 1,000 m.

Pumpkin

Pumpkin has long been known as a symbol of regeneration and longevity.

Muslim records hadith from the Prophet ﷺ who loved dried pumpkins and who said, " *Eat the pumpkin, it strengthens the intellect.*"[77]

The fleshy part of the pumpkin is rich in beta carotene and vitamin E. They are powerful antioxidants and are important for preventing and fighting cancer. Thanks to the cellulose contained in pumpkin, it has a purgative property, ie the ability to cleanse the body of harmful waste materials. Pumpkin is a good laxative and helps treat intestinal inflammatory changes and prevents cancer. It is also recommended for treating acne. The richness of naturally balanced vitamins and minerals in the tissues contributes to strengthening the body's resistance and for greater mental freshness and vitality.
Pumpkin seeds contain about 30% unsaturated fatty acids and are rich in minerals such as iron, zinc, phosphorus, and selenium, which are strong antioxidants.
The most important healing effect of the pumpkin seed oil is to improve prostate function. It is recommended to be used as an unrefined salad oil and to be often present in the diet of men.
Also, pumpkin seed oil enhances potency, accelerates postoperative recovery, and improves the general condition of the body. Snacking on pumpkin seeds provides many

healthy nutrients: protein, unsaturated fatty acids, fiber, vitamins, and minerals.

Incense

Enes, radiyallahu anhu, narrates the following hadith: *"Fill your homes with the scent of incense and thyme."* Abu Nuaym, radiyallahu anhu, reports that the Prophet ﷺ said: *"Give incense to your pregnant women because the male child that will be born will be strong and with a healthy heart, and if it is a female it will be attractive."*
It is no wonder that the Prophet Muhammad recommended incense before 1400. It is narrated in a hadith that a man complained to the Prophet ﷺ of forgetfulness so the Messenger of Allah ﷺ told him: *"Use incense because it heals the heart and gives him courage and is a cure for forgetfulness."* Ibn Abbas, may Allah be pleased with him, said that if we mix sugar and incense and eat it on an empty stomach we will have no problem with urination and amnesia.
Incense is of Arabic origin. The trunk of the tree is cut with a knife, from which the liquid drains. This liquid hardens despite the high temperature. Using a scraper, the hardened drops are collected. This is done once or twice a year. Different trees are used every year because the trees need time to recover. Today there are several plantations of this species. The more transparent and the less wood it contains the better. It contains pure liquid, water, rubber, essential oils, bitter ingredients, acids, plant traces, etc. So far, over 200 other chemicals have been found.
In Christianity, it is believed that incense is much more powerful than any other herb. Its intense scent instilled in people the belief that they could breathe again. Because it

was not available in large quantities, it became a luxury that enriched the church. Only in wealthy families did incense burn on coals. Incense became so popular that it became one of the most valuable gifts for the royal court. Its smoke was believed to ward off evil spirits. It was a concept familiar to the South American Indians. In some nations, it was known as a shield for travelers. Due to this and the paganisms that were made, many Muslims avoid incense even though it is mentioned as a medicine in the traditions of Muhammad ﷺ. Incense, unlike amber, was banned in ancient Judaism by the death penalty.

Today, with modern scientific methods, it has been determined that incense, as the Prophet Muhammad himself pointed out to us is a drug used to improve urination, for heart disease and as a cure for amnesia, ie. forgetfulness.

Pickles and compote

The Prophet practiced to use *nebiz* (pickle) as a drink that he made himself so that he pour clean water into a bowl, and then he put a handful of raisins, or dates, or almonds, etc. After 12 to 48 hours, he used it as a juice.

Today it is known in medicine that in this way special types of bacteria are formed, which are necessary for the proper functioning of the stomach system.

Everyone should take these bacteria into the body every day because they are very important for regulating metabolism. These bacteria are also found in liquid yogurt. It is interesting how we are neglecting the practice of Prophet ﷺ, and use artificial juices, which are the cheapest goods, to the point of paying for what harms our bodies.

Date

They are the "crown of sweets". The hadith of the Prophet says: "A house with dates does not feel hungry." [78]
Prophet sometimes combined dates with bread. Sometimes he mixed ripe dates and cucumbers or dates with liquid butter.
Dietitians consider dates to be the best food for women who need to give birth and those who are breastfeeding.[79] This is because dates contain elements that help alleviate maternal depression and enrich milk with all the elements necessary for a child to be healthy and resistant to disease. The Prophet stressed the importance of dates and their effectiveness in fetal growth. He also recommended that they are given to women.
While the date palm tree is called "nakhl," the fruit is called "tamr" in Arabic. The date palm, mentioned more than any other fruit-bearing plant in the Qur'an, is a symbol often associated with Islam and Muslims. Throughout the month of Ramadan, dates are a common ingredient in the Muslim diet.
The Prophet said: *"Break your fast by eating dates as it is purifying, "* (Ahmad).
Based on this Hadith, Muslims insist on breaking their fasts with dates. According to another Hadith, the Messenger said: *"Ajwah dates are from Paradise."* (Al-Tirmidhi)
Ajwah is one of the excellent varieties of dates grown in the Madinah region.
In Surah Maryam of the Holy Qur'an, Allah provided Prophet Isa's (peace be upon him) mother Maryam (peace be upon her) with fresh dates when she was experiencing discomfort and pain during the final stages of her pregnancy.
"Shake the trunk of the palm toward you and fresh, ripe dates will drop down onto you." (Surah Maryam, 25)

The significance of the date palm as a source of nutrition and sustenance is evident in the statement narrated by Ibn Umar (may Allah be pleased with him): *"The Prophet said there is a tree among the trees which is similar to a Muslim (in goodness), and that is the date palm tree."* (Bukhari)

In another hadith, the Prophet stressed the importance of dates as a major food item, saying, *"People in a house without dates are in a state of hunger."* (Muslim)

The excellence of date palms is also referred to in the following verse of the Holy Qur'an: ***"And in the earth are tracts (diverse though) neighboring, and gardens of vines and fields sown with corn, and palm trees — growing out of single roots or otherwise: watered with the same water, yet some of them We make more excellent than others to eat. Behold, verily in these things, there are signs for those who understand."*** (Surah Al-Raad, verse 4)

The date is also referred to in the Holy Qur'an as one of the blessings that would be offered in Paradise. In several traditions, the Prophet ate dates with some other fruits and vegetables. Abdullah ibn Jaafar, may Allah be pleased with him, said the *"Messenger ate cucumbers with dates."* (Al-Tirmidhi) According to two other traditions recorded by Al-Tirmidhi, the Prophet ate dates with watermelon or muskmelon.

The Prophet also taught his disciples that the date was not only an antidote to poison but also an effective defense against black magic. *"Whoever eats seven dates of the High Land of Madinah in the morning will not be hurt by poison or sorcery on that day."* (Bukhari)

In another Hadith, the Prophet exhorted the believers that *"you should defend yourselves from the hellfire even with a piece of date."*

Reference to the palm tree could also be seen in chapter Qaf, Al-Shuara and Al-Nahl of the Holy Qur'an. In early descriptions of the Prophet's Mosque in Madinah, historians state that the leaves of the date palm were used as a roof covering.

Dates contain natural sugar that is easily absorbed and digested, so it is safe and healthy for the stomach and intestines of children. The juice of dates is especially useful if you mix with milk which becomes even more nutritious and renewing drink for children and adults. A mixture of dates and honey is used to treat diarrhea and dysentery in children but should be taken three times a day.

This mixture also strengthens the gums during tooth growth. Here we should mention the tradition of the Prophet ie rubbing the gums of the newborn[80] with well-chewed dates and feeding on them. Science has confirmed that giving sugar dissolved in water provides the child[81], the newborn with the necessary nutrition, and improves their immunity.

Because we know that the sugar in dates is the most easily absorbed and digested, so it is most suitable for feeding newborns, but the date should be well chewed or soaked in water to be easier for the newborn to receive. Also dr. Enes er-Ravi claims that the child is born 100% sterilized, aseptic and that it lacks fluoride. This proves that the Prophet Muhammadﷺ surpassed today's doctors in this way of feeding. Dates are used for digestive and intestinal problems and also help to perform their function more effectively. They are also used for constipation. They should be soaked in water overnight and consumed the next morning after making a nice syrup.

The syrup from dates serves as a cure for the faint of heart. As well as for the treatment of sexual exhaustion. When mixed with milk and honey, dates can serve as a tonic for the treatment of sexual impotence for both sexes, and such syrup strengthens the body and raises energy levels. The elderly will also benefit from this syrup because it improves the condition and frees the body from toxins accumulated in the cells over the years. Strangely, Western doctors who treat their patients through fasting advise them to use the natural sugar contained in fruits and water when they break their fast. Thus, dates and water are the best food for the fasting person. Let us recall the hadith of the Prophet ﷺ: *"If you have a date, break your fast with it, if you don't have it, break the fast with water as it is purifying." (Abu Dawood)"* [82] .

The advise of the Prophet in such consumption of dates may be because the reduction of the feeling of hunger and consequently the reduction of the amount of food consumed; thus, fasting would be effective and beneficial. And if you remember that fasting is the best weapon to expel toxins from the body, then eating dates (*toxin - restive*) upon completing fasting is the most effective treatment against weakness and exhaustion as a result of an accumulation of toxic chemicals and heavy metals in cells in body.

Dates lose 1/3 of their water content when dried in the sun. Dried dates contain a high percentage of natural sugar, hence they are the best food for the fasting person. The wide variety of nutrients in dates makes them full. When we know that the cause of obesity is the constant feeling of hunger and appetite for food that makes a person consume larger amounts of fat and sugar. Dates will provide the body with the necessary sugar and stimulate the intestines, which reduces hunger and food consumption. We can conclude that dates can be used as an anti-obesity treatment. Also sipping juice dates used in the treatment of sore throat, various types of fever, nose runs and cold.

Dates are a great remedy for alcohol overdose. In such cases, drinking water in which fresh dates are crushed or soaked brings immediate relief. Let us mention one of the hadiths of the Prophet: *" Whoever eats 7 squeezed dates in the morning will not be able to be affected by magic or poisoning that day. "* [83]

Dear believer, if you feel weak, do not hesitate but take 7 dates in the morning as recommended by the Prophet ﷺ. These seven dates weigh about 70 grams, so if you take them you automatically receive 70 mg of calcium which is good for bones, joints, and nerves, 35 mg of phosphorus which is food for the brain and 7 mg of iron which strengthens the body as a whole and especially the heart. They are also suitable for weight loss because they contain 0.25 g of fat. So, if you are suffering from obesity, then this meal is suitable for you. This food regulates and stimulates the work of the intestines through 10 g of dietary fiber that it contains.

Dietary Institutes today recommend dates for children who are nervous or hyperactive. Modern science has also proven the effectiveness of dates in preventing diseases of the respiratory system. Aisha r.a., the wife of the Prophet ﷺ, recommended dates for those who suffered from dizziness. It is well known that low blood sugar and low blood pressure are among the causes of dizziness.

Dates also maintain eye health. They are very useful against night blindness. In the early years of Islam, dates served as food for Muslim fighters. They carried them in special bags hung on the side. They are the best muscle stimulant, and thus the best food for a fighter who has just entered a battle.

Black Seed (Nigella Sativa)

The Prophet said: *"The black cummin[86] contains a cure for every disease except death. "*[87]

The Nigella Sativa shell looks like a poppy shell, contains dark grains, which are dried after harvest. From these cold-pressed seeds, an oil-rich in unsaturated fatty acids is obtained. These acids are essential (vital), so with the food, they need to be absorbed into the body. Let's list just a few of the many diseases against which this miracle drug is used: for acne, allergies, and asthma, bloating, cellulite, colds, joint pain, lack of concentration, kidney stones, partial impotence, severe forms of infertility, gingivitis, cancer, and AIDS. Today is grown mainly in Syria, Iraq, Egypt, America, India, Pakistan, Iran, Greece and Cyprus because it thrives best in sunny areas.

The precious properties of black cumin have been known for a long time, so it is used in many cultures all over the globe. The seed of the black cumin (Latin: *Nigella Sativa*) is mentioned in the Bible under the name cumin. In ancient times, this seed was used to make bread. A bottle of black cumin oil is known to have been found in Tutankhamun's tomb. Pharaoh's doctors used this oil and black cumin cream in diseases of the digestive system.

 It was widely used in cosmetics; Nefertiti and Cleopatra cherished their body with oil flawed and used as an additive in a bath. Also, in the Orient, black cumin has been used for thousands of years to treat allergies and inflammation. Commonly used in asthma, bronchitis, and atopic. In ancient Greece, black cumin was known as a means of strengthening the physical and mental weakness of the sick. The tincture of black cumin oil has long been used in our region to treat bloating, diseases of the stomach, chest, liver, and much more. In Europe, this plant gained great popularity in the Middle Ages, after in 1031 writing of Ibn Sina was published in the *Book of Healing the Soul*.[88] Ibn Sina, among other things, describes the extraordinary action of the black cumin for maintaining health. Besides, the book contains numerous tips and recipes, which doctors still often recommend to their patients.

In the past decade, scientists from renowned research institutes (among others in the Center for Cancer Research *Hilton Head Island* in South Carolina) begin using modern methods, to analyze black cumin. The following results were obtained:

- The seeds of black cumin contain more than a hundred ingredients and positively affect health, encourage digestion, and work intestine.
- The substances in the black cumin extract strengthen the immune system in the fight against tumors.
- Black cumin oil acts against bacteria and fungal diseases.
- Black cumin oil has the effect of lowering blood sugar.
- The prolonged use of black cumin oil strengthens the immune system.

Also, they found that Nigella Sativa - extract, used in large quantities, causes the following:

- Stimulation of bone marrow cells (increase by 250%).
- Increased production of T - cells helpers and B - cells producing antibodies in the immune system.
- Retirement age production of interferon - proteins important for the immune system.
- Prevents the growth of cancer cells (50% growth retardation)

Another research institute, *Cancer Immuno - Biology Laboratory*, regardless of these results, experimented on animals and also found that chiropractic reduced the growth of cancer cells.

Unsaturated fatty acids, which are contained in chiropractic, are needed as key substances in tissue hormones. They stimulate metabolism and digestion. Also, they regulate cholesterol and enable healthy metabolism. So for hair and skin are of great importance.

A study in the Children's University Clinic in Minnesota showed that Gamma-linolenic slope acid contained in black cumin has an anti-asthmatic effect because it prevents allergic reactions. With increased stress, consumption of means for enjoyment, little exercise, the one-sided or wrong diet, we destroy our immune system. Modern immunological studies confirm that regular use of turmeric oil has a preventive effect against social diseases such as lung cancer, colon, and lymphatic cancer, clogged arteries, rheumatic diseases, the appearance of retinal detachment.

Long-term, consistent use of turmeric oil corrects the various symptoms of those who have had allergies in 90% of cases. Moreover, it enhances immune effects, helps allergy to pollen and dust in atopic, infections, and other diseases. Black cumin oil can be used as a dietary supplement up to 3 grams per day. It is the opinion of Dr. Peter Schleicher[89] from the Munich Department of Immunology.

It is important to know that the complete effect of the therapy comes only after 8 to 12 weeks of regular consumption, says the immunological expert Dr. Schleicher. The seeds of this growth are eaten either whole or mixed with honey, ie as oil obtained by compression or cooking.[90] *Nigella sativa* seeds contain essential oils, proteins, alkaloids, and soaps.

The many active ingredients in Nigella sativa are effective against many cancers, such as blood cancer: leukemia,[91] intestinal cancer, [92] skin cancer,[93] pancreatic cancer,[94] fibro-sarcoma,[95] prostate cancer,[96] breast cancer,[97] and others.

Pharmacologically important components of Nigella sativa extract have also been studied against lung cancer as an anticancer agent.[98]

One such study demonstrated the anti-tumor activity of α - Catherine extracted from Nigella sativa against Lewis lung cancer in experimental mice. The protective function of Nigella sativa extract induced oxidative stress, inflammatory response, and carcinogenesis of lung cells has also been demonstrated.[99]

These studies, together with in vitro study of cytotoxic activity of the extract from the seeds of Nigel Sativa and[100] indicate that they have a high cytotoxic effect. The great effect shown in laboratory tests indicates that Nigella Sativa significantly reduces the spread of cancer and that with a certain dosage can help as a cytostatic. A particularly strong effect is with the use of organic honey, which increases the in vitro abilities of Nigel and Sativa molecules. The best effect is achieved by taking Nigella honey and oil in the morning and evening on an empty stomach, in the ratio of one teaspoon of oil with half a teaspoon of honey, while at noon it is desirable to use honey mixed with freshly ground seeds instead of Nigella Sativa oil. Of course, to win the battle against cancer, it is not enough just to use this diet, but you need a therapy that primarily begins with spiritual purification and peace, using healthy fruit foods (grapes, melons, watermelons, pomegranates, bananas, apples, etc.) and vegetables (cauliflower, kale, spinach, garlic, etc.), avoiding harmful habits such as smoking, eating fatty, spicy foods, avoiding dairy products, complete elimination of crystallized sugars and refined oils, detoxification of the body, use of various teas, oil extracts as well as means of boosting immunity and the like.

Citrus (Lemon, Orange)

It is narratedin a reliable narration that the Messenger of Allah, may Allah peace him grant and him bless said:

"The example of a believer, who recites the Qur'an and acts on it, is like an orange (utrujjah) which tastes nice and smells nice. And the example of the believer who does not recite the Qur'an but acts on it is like a date that tastes

sweet but has no smell. And the example of the hypocrite who recites the Qur'an is like sweet basil which smells good but tastes bitter. And the example of a hypocrite who does not recite the Qur'an is like a colocynth (bitter apple) which tastes bitter and has a bad smell.". "[101]

Imam Al-Hafiki claimed that cedar-wood could be used to treat hemorrhoids. Lemon, orange, and cedar are an excellent source of vitamin C and a good source of vitamin A. These two vitamins stimulate the immune system and provide protection.

Lemon is full of antioxidants and plays a key role in energy production in the human body. Rich in nutrients, it tastes great and is low in calories. Lemon with its refreshing juice is a good addition to any diet. It makes you feel full and has few calories. It helps directly in the loss of calories and also helps to reduce the level of insulin in the blood.

Red lemon contains more antioxidants than ordinary lemon, so this may be the reason for their beneficial effect on triglycerides. Scientists recommend that all those who suffer from elevated levels of the cholesterol in the blood, be sure to include one red lemon per day in the diet.

Saffron

Saffron is warm and dry. It strengthens the heart and soul. Et Tirmizi reports that the Prophet recommends saffron and olive oil as a remedy for pleurisy.[102] Because saffron stimulates the sex, Prophet forbade wearing clothes dyed with saffron during Ramadan and pilgrimage. It is used as an ointment to treat itching and cracking of the skin. Today, modern science has studied the uses of saffron in detail.

Saffron is an extremely highly prized spice, used almost everywhere in the world. Although saffron is commonly used as a spice in cooking various dishes, it is an herb with many healing properties. Saffron crocin, saffron, and picrocrocin have anticancer properties that stop the growth of cancer cells in cancer patients. Saffron tea is used to treat depression. Studies have shown that consuming large amounts of this tea, but also the spice itself, reduces depression, and creates a feeling of happiness. Improves circulation and strengthens the heart.

In Chinese medicine, saffron is traditionally used to improve blood circulation and to treat bruises. The active ingredient crocin can also lower the concentration of cholesterol and triglycerides in the blood, thus preventing the development of atherosclerosis and the complications it can cause (heart attack, stroke, etc.). Rich in antioxidants, Saffronal, which is an integral part of saffron, is a powerful antioxidant and destroys free radicals, which can lead to cell and tissue damage.

Studies have shown that saffron improves eyesight and successfully prevents or alleviates macular degeneration, which is the most common cause of blindness in the elderly.

Milk

Surely there is a lesson for you in the cattle: We provide you to drink out of that which is in their bellies between the feces and the blood - pure milk which is a palatable drink for those who take it. (Quran, 16:66)

There are 4 parts of the belly which processes the excretion. And simultaneously it processes the production of milk. And finally, it is passed to the udder.

"Between excretions and the blood". This refers to the most wonderful process of the formation of pure milk in the bellies of the cattle. For, the fodder they eat turns into blood, filth, and pure milk, which is altogether different from the first two in its nature, color, and usefulness. Some cattle produce milk in such abundance that after suckling their young ones a large quantity of it is left to make excellent human food. To produce milk, cows need to eat a variety of grasses, clover, and bulky fodder, plus food that's rich in protein and energy.

It is known fact that Muhammad ﷺ loved milk. It is narrated from Ibn Masud r.a. that the Prophet ﷺ said:

"*Indeed, Allah did not give any disease without prescribing a cure except for old age. Therefore, drink cow's milk because the cow grazes on all kinds of herbs. *" And in another version, it says " *..in cow's milk is a cure for every disease. *"

Scientists from the University of Maine in the US, in a recent study, pointed out that taking a glass of milk every day improves almost all functions of the human organism, especially the brain. The study goes so far as to conclude that people who regularly consume milk have 5 times better results on memory tests than people who do not consume milk at all. Scientists add that the elderly should consume milk regularly. Apart from the other health benefits that milk offers, people who consume it will maintain good brain function for a long time in old age. Milk and dairy products are undoubtedly very healthy to use, except for people who due to other health problems should not use them. It has long been known that milk contains a significant amount of calcium, specific proteins, vitamin D, magnesium and other ingredients that play a role in preventing diabetes, protect bones and prevent obesity, and today we add the positive effect of milk on the work of the brain. So if we summarize all this, we can say with certainty that we must not forget and include diary product from birth to the end of life.

You can include milk in your daily diet in many ways, you can consume only a glass of milk in the morning or add it to your morning coffee, include it in a meal or similar. Yogurts are dairy products that may provide the most benefits for organism, so the daily use is always welcome.

Meat

Almighty Allah tells us: " *He makes you use the sea, eat fresh meat from it, and take out the ornaments with which you adorn yourselves ....* " [104]

Abu Hurairah narrated a hadith from the Prophet ﷺ *"Eating meat refreshes the heart."* [105]

One of the most used meats is beef. People often think that red meat is not part of a healthy diet, but research shows that if the intake of saturated fats is controlled and if meals containing red meat are properly balanced, it can be included in a heart-protective diet.

The Prophet told us: *"Chew the meat well because then it is more nutritious and easier to digest."* [106]

For scientific support of this claim of the Prophets, it is not required to argue.[107] Meat is rich in protein, and the body needs more energy to process these proteins than it needs for carbohydrates and fats. This means that the more protein you consume, the more your body works, so in the process, you burn more calories.

Studies show that people on a high-protein diet burn twice as many calories a few hours after eating as people on a high-carbohydrate diet.

The best way to reduce your risk of heart disease is to eat fish. Due to the high presence of omega 3 fatty acids in fish, it has been proven that it can prevent and treat many cardiovascular diseases. Statistics show that all over the world, people who frequently use fish in their diet are much less likely to develop heart or vascular disease. A Dutch study has shown that eating just 30 grams of fish a day can reduce the risk of heart attack by 5 %. If we could look inside the arteries in humans, we could see that the healthiest people are those who use fish in their diet daily, even in very small quantities. This was recently done by a group of Danish students, which confirmed the positive side of fish in the diet and its contribution to preventing the occurrence of atherosclerosis.

Danish scientists have received 40 samples of arteries taken from autopsies made at Frederic's Burke Hospital. They measured the fish oil in the adipose tissue, which showed which of the people used the fish in their diet. Undoubtedly the most permeable and cleanest were the blood vessels of the persons in whom the largest amount of omega 3 fatty acids was found in the adipose tissue, ie. people who often used fish in their diet.

The quail and its meat are mentioned as food that God sent down to the Israelis. Quail meat and eggs are a well-known remedy that is especially used for diseases of the lungs and airways.

Honey

Allah says in the Qur'an in the chapter An Nakhl (Bee):

"And your Lord taught the honey bee to build its cells in hills, on trees, and in (men's) habitations; Then to eat of all the produce (of the earth), and find with skill the spacious paths of its Lord: there issues from within their bodies a drink of varying colors, wherein is healing for

men: verily in this is a Sign for those who give thought. (
An-Nahl (The Bee), 68-69)

It is generally known that honey is a fundamental food source for the human body, whereas only a few people are aware of the extraordinary features of its producer, the honeybee.

As known, the food source of bees is nectar, which is not possible to be found during winter. For this reason, they combine the nectar collected in the summertime with special secretions of their body, produce a new food substance, which is honey, and store it for the coming winter months.

It is noteworthy that the amount of honey stored by the bees is much more than their actual need. The question which comes to the mind is why this "excessive production", which seems to be a waste of time and energy is not stopped? The answer to this question is hidden in the verse which states that the bee is "taught" by the Lord.

Bees innately produce honey not only for themselves but also for human beings. Bees, like many other beings in nature, are offered to the service of man. Just like the chicken laying at least one egg a day although it does not need it, or the cow producing much more milk than its offspring needs.

It is superfluous to speak of the benefits of honey. Honey is given by God as something good for man. Honey, royal jelly, pollen, propolis, and bee venom have been found to cure many diseases. It is a medicine that has been used for a long time. It is also interesting to note that Hippocrates discovered that honey and water were ideal for healing wounds. Honey is even used to treat patients who have a retinal detachment. Propolis helps treat many diseases such as skin problems, sexually transmitted diseases, and many other disorders. [109]

This precious wealth and heritage include the traditions of the Prophet's medicine, his instructions on how to face and protect one of Allah's greatest blessings to man, health. All doctors agree that honey is the most useful medicine for humans because it contains disinfectants, strengthens the body and stomach, and improves appetite. It is useful for the elderly and those with increased blood pressure.

It is narrated that the Prophet, ﷺ, said: "I recommend two medicines: honey and the Qur'an."

The Prophet ﷺ also said: "If there is any good in your medicines, then it is hijamah (discharge of harmful blood from the human body) and honey."[110]

Honey contains great benefits, cleanses harmful substances in the veins, intestines, and helps other organs. It is reported that a man came to the Prophet ﷺ and he said: *"My brother complains of the stomach pain.",* and in another front reads: *"is stricken with dysentery."* The Prophet ﷺ said: *"Give him honey."* The man left, but after a day he came back and said: *"I gave him, but nothing helped."* In another tradition he said: *"The disease only worsened.",* so two or three times and each time the Prophet said: *"Give him to eat honey.",* and the third or fourth time the man said that he is healed. Prophet said: *"Allah told the truth and the belly of your brother lied (at the start of the infection). "* [111]

It is reported that the Prophet on an empty stomach drank a glass of honey mixed with water. Honey is more effective in fighting infections than antibiotics without causing side effects. When honey and water mix, the properties of honey doubles. This is because a chemical reaction takes place and as a result, a hydrogen factor is created - the most powerful natural antibiotic. If you decide to try a natural recipe for good health, a glass of warm water, and a teaspoon of honey in the morning is enough. Experiments performed with honey show that its bactericidal properties are doubled when diluted with water. It only takes seven minutes for the mixture of water and honey to penetrate the bloodstream and begin to fight infections.

Because honey sugar molecules can be converted to other sugars (ie fructose to glucose), despite its high acidity, honey is easily digested by people with the most sensitive stomachs. It helps the kidneys and intestines to function better. It has a low caloric value. The quality of honey is seen compared to the same amount of sugar - it gives the body 40% fewer calories. Although honey gives the body a lot of energy, it does not increase its weight. Free sugar molecules of honey improve brain function because the brain is the largest consumer of sugar.

Honey provides an important part of the energy that the body needs to build blood cells. Therefore, it helps purify the blood. Honey has certain positive effects in regulating and improving blood circulation. It also acts as protection against capillary problems and arteriosclerosis. Destroys bacteria. This bactericidal property of honey is called the "inhibitory effect". Royal jelly is a substance that bees produce in the hive. This nutrient contains sugar, protein, fat, and many vitamins. The highest quality of honey is spring honey, then summer and winter honey. Different types of honey often act on specific ailments. For example, linden and sage honey relieve respiratory problems and colds, but linden honey is not recommended for heart patients. Lavender honey is used against bloating and regulates heart function, helps with stomach ulcers, improves urination, and also works against tension or migraines. Dark chestnut honey stimulates circulation, regulates the work of the stomach, intestines, liver, it is recommended for anemia (anemia), relieves fatigue and strengthens muscles, as well as the body's immunity. Acacia honey is used for problems with the vascular system, in prison, and because it has a calming effect, it also helps with insomnia, nervousness, and tension. Meadow (flower) honey is especially recommended for strengthening immunity.

Tightly closed, honey has an unlimited shelf life. At a temperature of 41 degrees Celsius, honey loses its healing properties, and when adding it to tea, care should be taken not to be too hot. Crystallized honey's natural function does not affect its quality. This unique golden liquid is a much healthier alternative to white sugar, so it improves and preserves your health with this sweet gift from God.

Olive tree

In the Qur'an 1400 years ago, the Almighty Creator addressed the people in the chapter Mu'minun with the following words:

And a tree (olive tree) that grows on Mount Sinai that gives oil and spice, and eat from it! (Mu'minun, 20)

Muhammad ﷺ said in a hadith narrated by Ibn 'Umar: "Use olive oil and rub with it because it is obtained from the blessed tree." The following hadith from Muhammad comes to us from Alkame ibn Amir ﷺ: *Every kind of olive is for you, so smear yourself with olive oil because it is a help for those who have problems with hemorrhoids."* This tradition is also recorded by Ibn Qayyim al-Jawzi.

The olive tree is an evergreen tree that grows to a height of 10 meters. It branches massively and irregularly and has a massive and complex root system. The leaves have quite short stalks, and their shape is elongated elliptical. Like any other fruit, this one is green at first and then ripens until it turns black. Olive fruit contains as much as 35% oil, which is not only a spice but also a natural remedy. Due to its beneficial properties, olive oil is also called "Mediterranean gold". It is interesting to note that the olive tree leaf also has extremely effective healing effects. The ingredients that can be found in the leaf are very specific and are used to make various remedies to lower blood pressure. You can also use the olive tree leaf in case of urinary tract problems and to facilitate urination. The leaf is harvested when it is fully developed and formed, and then it must be dried before anything can be made from it. There are many different specific substances in olive leaves, but the most important is the substance *oleuropein*. If you have the opportunity to acquire olive leaves, you can easily make tea from them that will be very useful for your blood vessels, especially if you have chronic hypertension. People who have practiced this tea say that it gives excellent effects in a much shorter time than other similar teas. Quality olive oil has a slightly bitter taste, greenish color, and has a fruity aroma. The heavy smell of olive oil is a sign of poor quality and outdated oil.

Virgin olive oil (olio Vergine) - the healthiest and highest quality olive oil, which is obtained with the first cold pressing of healthy olives, and the olive seed must not be compressed. During the squeezing procedure, the use of heat must not occur, so only the so-called "Cold squeezing". Virgin olive oil has less than 1% free fatty acids. Virgin olive oil is very healthy because it contains many useful nutrients, which are strong antioxidants. Therefore, olive oil is also prescribed anticancer properties.
Nutritionists consider extra virgin olive oil to be a portion of very healthy food, rich in chlorophyll, carotene, lecithin (a natural antioxidant that stimulates the metabolism of fats, sugars, and proteins), polyphenols (antioxidants) and essential vitamins D, E, and K.
Some studies have shown that olive oil helps breast cancer patients. Antioxidants polyphenols, found in cold-pressed

olive oil, reduce the effect of the HER2 gene, which affects the development of breast cancer, according to a study by a Spanish student. Scientists have established with certainty why Mediterranean foods, which are rich in fruits, vegetables, and olive oil, can help women prevent and treat breast cancer. [1]

Virgin olive oil is also used to treat gallstones and bile ducts. It is a very good natural remedy, which stimulates the secretion of bile. Butter oil can also be used to treat skin ulcers and is used in the form of heated compresses. Olive oil also helps with inflammation of the intestines or stomach. It is a mild cleanser that does not irritate the skin. However, it can also be used to treat bleeding hemorrhoids. Olive oil and garlic salad is a natural remedy rich in healing ingredients, vitamins, minerals, and the most useful fats. If you put 2 tablespoons of vinegar in a deciliter of olive oil, you will get an excellent natural means to prevent and alleviate sunburn. For rheumatic pains, various skin inflammations, and itching, olive oil massage is very effective.

Today's science and scientific research confirm all these legends and words which is proof of the supernatural knowledge that Muhammad had ﷺ 1400 years ago.

Myrtle

Myrtle (*Myrtus munis*) is a plant that originates from the east of the Mediterranean, and has been transferred since prehistoric times. It blooms from April to August with

---

[1] Dr. Javier Menendez from the Catalan Oncology Institute and Dr. Antonio Segura Carretero of the University of Granada, examining which ingredients are most effective against breast cancer, found that quality unrefined olive oil contains a number of "phytochemical" ingredients that can cause malignant cell death.

white and soft scented flowers with 5 petals. The fruits are berries, which ripen in November. It is growing in wild Mediterranean areas because it is mild and warm.

 It helps in the treatment of digestive problems, intestinal diseases, bladder diseases, gum treatment, the lining of the mouth and tongue as well as disorders of the rectum of the uterus. If we smell it, it will reduce our headache. Myrtle is benefiting in empowering to stop bleeding and destroy bacteria. It also strengthens the organs. The Arabs use myrtle as a fragrant plant. The Prophet said: *"If anyone offers you Myrtle as a gift, do not turn it down. "It is from the Gardens of Paradise."*[2]

Myrtle syrup can also be made, but will not be used unless mixed with quince. Ibn Abbas r.a. has said, " *When Noah left the Ark, the first plant he planted was myrtle."*

He also mentions the narration in which he says: *"Adam a.s. has left heaven with three things: myrtle - queen of all fragrant plants on earth, thick date - queen of all date palms on earth, corn stalk - queen of all food in the world. "*[3]

The blessed effect of water on our health

The Prophet said: *"The most beautiful drink in this world and the next is water."* He also added: *" A man who will give water to his wife to drink has a reward for it.*

" El-Irbad said:*" I came to my wife and gave her water. I conveyed what I heard from the Prophet.*[4]

Water is essential for life. Humans can survive much longer without food than without water. The only thing we need

---

[2] Dželaluddin Abdurrahman es-Sujuti, *Vjerovjesnikova medicina*, Libris, Sarajevo, 2003., стр.71-72.
[3] Hadith from Ebu Nuaim.
[4] Ahmed, No. 16529.

for life more than water is air. Water represents about 60-70% of our body weight. Therefore, every part of our body needs it to function properly. Insufficient water intake leads to dehydration, in which case the normal functioning of the body is impossible. Even mild dehydration immediately has negative consequences such as decreased energy, headaches, fatigue.

Water is essential for life, but also for maintaining health and maintaining good look.

Water speeds up metabolism, increases energy levels, moisturizes the skin, and helps the body get rid of harmful toxins. Here are some of the benefits that drinking water brings us for better health and a more attractive appearance.

Water increases energy. One of the most common reasons people feel tired during the day is dehydration. Even the slightest dehydration leads to a decrease in energy. Water helps the blood to transport oxygen and other substances to different cells in the body. When the body has enough water, the energy level is higher.

Water helps in weight loss. That is why every diet recommends drinking at least 2 liters of water a day. Consuming 1-2 glasses of water before a meal significantly reduces appetite and leads to lower calorie intake. But, besides, water speeds up the metabolism, especially if it is cold. When you consume cold water, the body tries to warm up, and to do so, it consumes extra calories as well.

Water helps you exercise better and longer. Water regulates body temperature during exercise. If you drink enough water, you will have more energy and strength to complete the exercise. Besides, water will help prevent muscle cramps. Therefore, drink plenty of water before exercise, during exercise, and after physical activity.

Water improves digestion. Fiber and water are a strong combination that improves digestion. In contrast, dehydration causes the body to absorb all the water, leaving the colon dry, thus complicating the defecation process.

Water reduces the risk of kidney stones. Experts warn that frequent cases of kidney stones in children and adults are a consequence of insufficient water consumption. Water dissolves minerals and salts in the urine that contribute to the formation of stones. Drink enough water to significantly reduce the likelihood of kidney stones.

Water reduces stress and increases concentration. Given the fact that about 80% of our brain weight is water, then it is not difficult to assume that dehydration is an obstacle to its normal functioning. Lack of water causes stress to both body and mind and also reduces the ability to concentrate.

Water can cure headaches. Headache often occurs as a consequence of dehydration. In that case, consuming a few glasses of water will help you get rid of the unpleasant pain.

Water fights wrinkles and acne. Think of water as a natural remedy that nourishes your skin in different ways. When the body is dehydrated, fine lines and wrinkles are more visible. Water improves circulation, so your skin will get a healthy glow.

Water is crucial for body hygiene and human health. Start using the power of the water that Allah has given us right now.

The Prophet said, *"The key to paradise is prayer, and the key to prayer is purity."* Ibn 'Umar narrates that the Messenger ﷺ said: *"Prayer is not accepted without ritual washing (ablution) before prayer."*

Ibn Abbas r.a reports that the Prophet ﷺ said: *"I have to wash before performing the prayer."*

Almighty Allah has commanded: ***"O you who have believed when you rise to [perform] prayer, wash your faces and your forearms to the elbows and wipe over your heads and wash your feet to the ankles."***[5]

---

[5] Quran, Al-Ma'ida, 6;

Washing with water helps fight stress, nervousness, reduces the negative consequences of an event. Bad habits can be washed off with water. Scientists have found that washing the head, rinsing the face, and even simply washing the hands helps to get rid of negative emotions. All we have to do is put our hands under running water or take a shower and our bad memories will disappear. It has been established that in some cases even the mere thought of washing or bathing can help a person get rid of negative emotions, bad feelings, as well as eliminate doubt in the correctness of some choices.

Physical removal of dirt creates an association for the removal of mental dirt as well. Interestingly, in many ancient rituals, water was used as a catalyst, and even modern psychologists consider and recommend washing the face several times during the day, especially after surviving something unpleasant. This was pointed out to us by the Prophet who gave us advice that when we are angry it is desirable to take ablution.

In the Sunnah books,[6] Prophet said: *"Anger (wrath) comes from Satan. Satan is created from fire, and the fire is extinguished by water. So when one of you gets angry, let him perform ablution."*

The miracle of Zemzem water

Unusually, the spring of Zemzem[7] runs among solid, crystallized eruptive rocks more than 3000 years, despite all the excavations and encumbering that have occurred in its interior and around it. The daily flow of water is between 11 and 18.5 liters per second. This source of

---

[6] Abu Dawud, Ahmed, Abd al-Razak and At Tabarani. Reliable and well-known collections of narrations.

[7] The source is located next to the Kaaba.

information was not known until the time when tunnels were dug around Mecca. The workers noticed that the water was spilling through the cracks that spread over a greater distance in all directions around Mecca.

Groundwater is naturally carbonated mineral water. It consists of minerals that have a total of 2000 mg / l and thus the water is rich in minerals. The groundwater per liter contains 200 mg of calcium and 50 mg of magnesium. Zemzem is one of the heavy water and today scientific research shows that heart disease is less common in places where people drink heavy water.

Zemzem is an obvious miracle that emphasizes the dignified status of the Prophet Ibrahim (Abraham, peace be upon him), the father of the Prophet Ismail a.s. , who helped him build the Kaaba, and his truthful mother Hager (Agara).

It is reported that the mother of the believers Aisha r.a., it was her customary that every time she visited Mecca to bring Zemzem water to Medina, and so did the Prophet. They gave this water to the sick.[120] He poured it on their bodies and they, by the will of Allah, were healed.

The prayer of Ibrahim a.s. consisted of the following words: "Our Lord, I have settled some of my descendants in a place where nothing is sown, at Your Holy Temple, our Lord, to perform the prayer; therefore make the hearts of some people yearn for it and supply them with various fruits to be grateful.[121]

The Messenger of God told in numerous hadiths about the benefits of Zemzem water. Thus Ibn Abbas r. a. conveys that the Messenger of God said: "The best water on earth is the Zemzem. It is food for the hungry and medicine for the sick. Dzabir r.a. conveys that the Messenger of God has said: "Water is a service for what it will be used for.[122]

Japanese scientist Dr. Mesaru Emoti[123] claimed that Zemzem has special properties and characteristics that are not found in ordinary water. Emoto's book *The Hidden*

Messages in Water published in 2004 was a New York Times bestseller. This Japanese writer, the founder of the theory of `Crystallization of water atoms`, published several volumes of this work, which contain photographs of ice crystals and accompanying experiments.

After his long research on Zemzem water, he acknowledges that mixing one drop of Zemzem water with 1000 drops of plain water gives a mixture that has the same properties and characteristics as Zemzem water. Dr. Mesaru Emoti also pointed out that during the experimentation he put on cassettes of learning the Qur'an near the Zemzem water and this affected it and led to the conversion of the crystal-shaped form of the water. The water was perfectly clean and glowing, and he added that this was the strangest event to him during his exploration of Zemzem water.

He added that Zemzem water has the characteristic of 'remembering',[125] that is, retaining data within oneself, so for example if one were to study a chapter (surah) of the Qur'an at Zemzem water, later technology could reveal which chapter (surah) it was, by creating special Waves of the Zemzem water during the voice of the Qur'an, invisible to the naked eye.

Health and hygiene in Islam

Bathing

The human body is estimated to be home to 100 trillion bacteria. Many of them play an important role in maintaining physiological functions, including the development of the immune system, aiding in metabolic processes, and maintaining good health.

It is also recommends bathing on various occasions. That is a proof of Islamic consistency in terms of cleanliness and hygiene. Abdullah b. Omer r.a., reports that Prophet said:

"When any of you goes to Jumu'ah (Friday prayer), let him take a bath!"

Abu Said Al-Khudri reports: *"I bear witness that God's messenger (peace be upon him) said: 'Taking a bath on Friday is a duty on everyone who has attained puberty, as is cleaning his teeth and wearing some perfume if he finds it'."* (Reported by Al-Bukhari).

The great majority of scholars are of the view that taking a bath or shower on Friday is strongly recommended, before going out to attend the Friday prayer, which must be offered in congregation. The Prophet also recommended us to use a toothbrush to clean our teeth and mouths. This would ensure that no one will have a bad mouth smell when they come to the mosque. Also, he has recommended us to wear some perfume.

It is known that after intimate intercourse, the pores of our skin become quite clogged, so bathing after that contributes to the cleansing of those pores, dirt, and sweat. There is a wisdom of gusul for human hygiene, especially bathing after intimate intercourse, which over time, science will prove. Hence, Islam encourages bathing in various forms, as a kind of prevention against dirt and meeting high hygiene standards. When this encouragement was so pronounced at a time when there was a shortage of water, one can imagine what the recommendation of Islam would be in our conditions, when we have abundant water, when we have various possibilities for its heating and comfortable baths.

All this should be followed by environmental awareness in water consumption.

It is a well-known Hadith that says that one should not overdo washing, but use as much water as is enough to wash.

The Prophet was passing by Saad who was performing ablution and he told him: *"Do not overdo it with water."* Saad told, *" We can exaggerate with the use of the water?"* The Prophet said, "Yes, even if you are on the bank of a river ."[127]

Of course, this suggests that there should be environmental awareness. This was pointed out to us by a man who lived 1400 years ago, while human civilization today strives for maximum water saving. And Allah is the Guide of the hearts.

Islam toilet etiquette

Islamic toilet etiquette is a set of personal hygiene rules in Islam followed when going to the toilet. This code of Muslim hygienic jurisprudence is known as Qadaa' al-Haajah.

The main necessity of the Qur'an is washing one's hands and face with pure earth if the water isn't accessible.

While on the latrine, one must stay quiet. Talking, answering greetings, or welcome others is firmly debilitated. While defecating together, two men can't converse, nor take a look at one another's privates. Eating any food while on the latrine is strictly illegal.

The rear-end must be washed with water utilizing the left hand with an odd number of smooth stones/rocks called jamrah or hijaarah,(Sahih Al-Bukhari 161, Book 4, Hadith 27) subsequent to defecating. It is currently more normal to wipe with tissues and furthermore use water. So also, the penis or vulva must be washed with water with the left hand subsequent to urinating.

When leaving the latrine, one is encouraged to leave with the correct foot, and state a petition – "Praise is to Allah who relieved me of the filth and gave me relief.

Hand washing

Washing hands before and after eating it is Sunnah[128] , as stated in the narration of Aisha r.a. In the tradition which transmits Abu Hurejre r.a. warned:*"The one who sleeps with oily hands of food, unwashed, so if something happens to him, let him not rebuke anyone but himself!"*

Dirty, germ-infected hands are crucial in transmitting the causes of intestinal, metabolic process, and skin infectious diseases. Washing your hands with soap is one among the foremost effective measures to prevent diarrhoea and respiratory illness, diseases that are most to blame for the death of kids up to the age of 5. Spreading the habit of washing hands with soap and heat water will considerably contribute to reducing sickness and mortality.

Research shows that individuals living in urban areas, mostly ladies, wash their hands often.

Doctors advise that hands mustn't be washed solely before ingestion and once they are visibly unclean, however conjointly once intake and going to the bathroom, touching the nose, mouth or eyes, contact with a diseased person, and additionally during daily activities within the family.

The soap with that you wash your hands should be washed underneath running water once and hold on so it'll be clean, It's is necessary to rub the complete surface of the skin on your hands with soup, because the doctors advocate.

Today, once science has reached the height of its progress and that clearly emphasizes that washing hands before and once ingestion may be an essential that has got to be respected, we have a tendency to conclude what Islam has delivered to humanity, eager to educate it, not solely in spiritual, but additionally the most common queries that mean life and health.

The Muslims took this recommendation seriously, and therefore the best-confirmed example is of imam Hanbal. Abu Bakr al-Maruzi says:*"I saw that I had Ahmed b.Hanbel washes his hands before and after eating, even though he did ablution before that !"* [129]

Eating with the right hand

Preferring the right side is one of the peculiarities of Islam, especially when it comes to consuming food and fluids.

Ibn 'Umar (may Allah be pleased with him) reported that the Messenger of Allah (may Allah's peace and blessings be upon him) said: "If anyone of you eats, let him eat with his right hand, and if he drinks, let him drink with his right hand, for indeed the devil eats with his left hand and drinks with his left hand."

Analyzing what the Prophet ﷺ said about Satan and his actions, we will find that he mentions him for everything that could have negative consequences for a man, not only when it comes to his spiritual, but also physical dimension. Logically, if his left hand is used to remove dirt while performing physiological needs, it might help the hygiene of a person, so the devil is the one who is an accomplice in every spiritual and physical illness. When we look at the Islamic moral norms, in this regard we can notice that the right hand is most often used for beautiful things, such as shaking hands with people, writing, reading, eating, drinking, while with the left-hand things seem unclean and undesirable, such as washing the nose, washing the genitals and pubic areas, removing impurities and the like. Islam has set boundaries and given direction in which the body should move and establish harmony with nature and other people.

Why is it not healthy to drink water standing up ?!

We have often heard older people say *do not drink water while standing*. The Prophet Muhammad ﷺ warned us not to drink standing water. He inform us about this thing that at first glance seems pointless, but when you read it better and think about it, you will see that these words have many benefits for our health. The following hadiths warn us about this. Muhammad ﷺ said:

"If people knew what harm they do to the stomach by drinking water while standing, they would immediately vomit what they drank."[131] Also on this topic, he Prophet ﷺ conveyed to us:

"Let none of you drink while standing, and if he drinks let him try to get it back."[132]

Science today confirms the wisdom behind this warning. But why not drink water while standing, what is the medical explanation?

The position of the stomach differs in sitting and standing position. The man who stands when he consumes water and liquid food it goes directly to the 12th thumb intestine. In the stomach itself there is a circular arc and the liquid food and water when it follows this continuous path comes out through a small opening in the stomach (pylorus) and enters the duodenum. If people were to drink water while sitting, it would collect in the stomach and kill all the microbes in it, and only then would it pass into the duodenum. In this case, people who drink water while sitting will be protected from many diseases, as well as cholera. People who drink juices while standing uncontrollably, are at the highest risk.

In this case, people who drink water while sitting will be protected from many diseases such as cholera.

Putting your hand in front of your mouth when sneezing

As early as fourteen centuries ago, the Messenger of Allah put his hand or clothes in front of his mouth when sneezing, showing how a Muslim should behave on that occasion.

Abu Hurairah (may Allah be pleased with him) narrated:

" The Messenger of Allah, may Allah bless him put his hand or clothes in front of his mouth while sneezing and thus silenced it " .

It was narrated from Saeed from his father, that Abu Hurairah radiyallahu 'anhu said: Allah's Messenger Sallallahu 'Alayhi wa Sallam said, 'Allah likes sneezing, and He dislikes yawning, so if one of you yawns, let him suppress it as much as he can, and not make any noise, for that comes from Shaitan who is laughing at him.' [Hadith No. 5028, Book of Etiquette, Sunan Abu Dawud, Vol. 5]

Ibn Hajar, interpreting this hadith, believes that the Prophet of Islam did it so as not to disturb any of his conversational partner and so that something from the mouth would not come out of the sneeze, which could have occurred to them. Today, when we know how contagious diseases can be transmitted by sneezing and cough, we conclude that the Prophet ﷺ acted with great wisdom.

Sneezing also helps to remove the disease from the body more easily.

Procedure in yawning. It's ugly and distasteful to see a person who yawns, and it seems inappropriate because of various grimaces, on the other hand, prevents him from holding the mouth open without protection, dust, bacteria, or something undesirable and harmful to enter the human body and infect it. Yawning is an act that we can not easily prevent. It is usually the result of insufficient sleep, excessive sleep, or overeating. God does not like yawning, because it causes laziness, and He loves sneezing because after him the person thanks to the Noble Allah, and thus, remembers Him. The natural act of sneezing is the mercy and grace of Allah. It relieves us from discomfort, and we should thank Allah 'azza wa jall for it. When you say "alhamdulillah" when you sneeze, you're reviving a sunnah!

Narrated Abu Hurairah radiyallahu 'anhu: Allah's Messenger said: 'If anyone of you sneezes, he (she) should say "Alhumdulillah" (Praise be to Allah) and his brother or his companion (i.e. one who is with him/her) should say ''Yarhamuk Allah'' (May Allah have mercy on you). When the latter says ''Yarhamuk Allah," the former should say ''Yahdikumullah, wa yuslihu balakum'' (May Allah guide you and set your affairs straight).' [Hadith No. 6224, Book of Al-Adab, Sahih Bukhari, Vol. 8]

Brushing your teeth in Islam

In addition to bathing, brushing your teeth is an act of personal hygiene. Prophet said: *"If i would not make it difficult for my ummah*[133] i *would order them to perform ablution for every prayer, and to brush their teeth with every ablution. "*[134]
Brushing your teeth or cleansing your gums[135] was the practice not only of our Prophet, but it was the practice of the other Prophets before him.

Abu Ayyub r.a. , reports that the Prophet ﷺ said: The four things are Sunnah [ie. practice.] and of former Prophets: shame, smell, use of the miswak [Special wood used for brushing teeth] and marriage [137] ! "

How much is the Prophet of Islam ﷺ took care of the hygiene of his teeth and mouth, the best confirmation of the legends of Aisha and Husayfe r.a .

In the narration of Aisha r.a., it is said that the Prophet ﷺ when entering the house, first cleaned his teeth with miswak, a narration in which the Huzejfe ra, says, " *When the Prophet woke, he rubbed the mouth with miswak!* "

The mouth is the entrance for food and liquid and, when traces of food or liquid remain in it, microbes that multiply quickly settle and because of them ugly smells prevail in the mouth, and the organic acids then destroy the tooth tooth enamel and occur of caries. It all causes gingivitis and various dental diseases.

So, teeth must be kept clean and by protecting the teeth we protect the whole body. Miswak is the best solution for all problems because it contains substances that are deadly to microbes. How much the Messenger of Allah, ﷺ, stressed this type of care, best illustrates the hadith that Abu Hurejra said.: " *If I did not make it difficult for my ummah - or the people - I would order them to use the miswak (brushing their teeth) before every prayer.* "[138]

In the time of Allah's Messenger ﷺ today's toothbrush was not known, nor they used toothpaste .[139]

Protection through eating and drinking

The human body needs to eat and drink. Food is an essential element for maintaining the human body. That is why we see how Islam commands the non-believer to eat permissible and beautiful things. Allah says:

"O you who believe, feed on the good things that We have provided for you, and be grateful to Allah if you serve Him."[141]

From that point of view, Islam forbids its followers certain things, and that is mainly because of their harmfulness. A

Muslim is strictly forbidden to consume alcohol, and a wise person is aware of its harmful effects and consequences.

Islam has also categorically forbidden the eating of pork because of its harmfulness to human health. Allah says in the Qur'an:

"He hath forbidden for you only carrion and blood and swine flesh and that immolated in the name of any other than Allah..."[142]

So basically everything that is forbidden to man is harmful, which is a great indicator of the perfection of Islam and its immense concern for human health.

Halal diet

Halal is an Arabic term meaning "permissible". In the context of nutrition, the term refers to food that is permissible under Islamic law.[143]

It is estimated that 70% of Muslims around the world follow this diet. For the less informed, "halal" is a food that is allowed under Islamic law, and in recent years has been widely consumed in more developed countries because it is considered a healthy food. In contrast, "haram" is food that is not allowed and is avoided by Muslims.

For an animal to come from a farm to a table, it is necessary from the very beginning to have a complete but healthy upbringing, to be well-fed, to be well treated, not to be harmed, and to be sacrificed according to Islamic law.

That also means that you need to eat clean food and water and not be fed with animal and harmful products. Consuming food that has not been treated with pesticides, toxins and other pollutants is a health benefit, not only for Muslims but for all people.

As "halal" food are considered:

- fish and seafood,
- eggs,
- milk,
- all kinds of fruits and vegetables,
- the meat of slaughtered animals to be by Islamic law (except for forbidden animals);
- beverages such as coffee, teas, juices, and other beverages and products that do not contain alcohol as an ingredient, but if they cause harm, it become prohibited.

The Qur'an forbids various substances as illegal, ie "haram" for consumption:
- Pork or any pork products (eg trotters, clothing, footwear pork ka leather, etc. (*Qur'an, 2: 173*)
- Blood (*Qur'an, 2:17*)
- Animals slaughtered in the name of anyone but God (*Qur'an, 2: 173*)
- Carcass (*Qur'an, 5: 3*),
- According to tradition - all carnivorous animals, except for fish and marine life.
- It is forbidden to consume all opioids (especially alcohol and narcotics). (*Qur'an, 2: 219*)

Muslims in Southeast Asia believe that animals that live both on land and in water (such as amphibians, some reptiles, and some species of birds) are not safe to eat. The snail-eating permit is valid for both land and sea snails. If they are cooked alive there is nothing wrong with that, because the earth snails have no blood, so it could be said that they do not have to be slaughtered, while the sea snails are provided with the general permissibility of sea catch and food.

The world market of halal products annually makes a turnover of 850 billion USD and is one of the fastest-growing markets in the world with a growth rate of 40% so far, and future growth is estimated at 50% per year. The economies of Saudi Arabia, Bahrain, the United Arab Emirates, Qatar, Oman, and Kuwait weigh $ 715 billion.[145] Countries in our environment are already entering these markets through the door by introducing the "halal" standard in their operations. Some years ago, Macedonia started distributing halal certificates.

Prohibition of pork

Islam categorically forbids eating pork because of its harmfulness to human health. Allah says in the Qur'an:

"Surely He has prohibited for you only carrion (i.e. dead meat) and blood and the flesh of swine, and whatever has been acclaimed to other than Allah. ... "[146]

It is similar in the Bible verse where is found in Deuteronomy: *"And you may not eat the pig. It has split hooves but does not chew the cud, so it is ceremonially unclean for you. You may not eat the meat of these animals or even touch their carcasses.."*[148] If a person touches anything unclean--whether the carcass of an unclean wild animal or livestock or crawling creature--even if he is unaware of it, he is unclean and guilty.

Let's see what bacon and fat do to your blood vessels? A sandwich luxuriously filled with bacon for breakfast is a real "delayed bomb" for your body, studies show. Researchers have found that a single full-fat meal can affect the health of your heart, so in people who eat pie or similar fatty foods in the early morning, the effects can be seen before lunch. Namely, fatty foods are associated with the occurrence of atherosclerosis - narrowing of the arteries. Fat can build up in the arteries. Consumption of pork causes many types of diseases. Eating pork can cause over seventy different types of diseases. The person can get various infectious parasites such as roundworm, needle worm, mining worm. One of the most dangerous is Taenia Solium, which is known as a parasite. It lives in the human intestine and is very long, that is, it can sometimes stretch along the small the small digestive tract. While this worm is in humans, it lays its infinitesimally little eggs, but the eggs enter the bloodstream of the body and thus can reach all parts of the body. If they enter the brain, then they can cause memory loss. If it enters the heart it can cause a heart attack, if it reaches the eye it can cause blindness, and in the liver, it can lead to damage to the liver itself. This bacterium in the form of a long thin worm can damage almost all organs of the body. Another dangerous parasite is Trichura Tichurasis.

A common misconception among people about pork is that if cooked well this parasite dies. A U.S.-based research project has found that of the 24 people who suffer from these parasites, 22 are those who have cooked pork for a long time. This directly indicates that these parasites present in the pork do not die at high temperatures while boiling or roasting.

Furthermore, the pig is one of the dirtiest animals on earth and lives in the mud, in it's feces. The pig is the best collector of waste and garbage. In the villages where there are no modern toilets, the villagers perform the physiological needs in the open, very often the pigs are the ones who clean the feces behind the villagers. A pig is an animal that eats its dead child, but can often eat a human corpse, if it reaches it.

The harmfulness of alcohol

The word "hamr" (wine) in Arabic means "to cover the vessel." It is said that this name was given cause alcohol covers and seduces the mind no matter what state it is in solid or liquid. Unlike this-worldly wine, another wine is mentioned in the Qur'an, and that is the wine of paradise, which has different characteristics and is devoid of any flaws and consequences for the mind and reason. Allah says: *"**There is no headache from it, nor is the intellect lost!**"*[149]

Paradise wine does not make you drunk and does not contain alcohol, it does not darken your mind, nor is there any harm. On the other hand, everything that intoxicates and destroys the human mind is marked as drunkenness. This is what Er Razi claims in *Mukhtar es Sihah*. Before the advent of Islam, the Arabs drunk large quantities of wine and feasted on it. At the same time, they gave special importance to the wine and sung about the wine, the glasses in which it was served, and the drinks they made. The reason why Islam forbade wine, alcohol, and everything obtained from various kinds of fruits (grapes, apples, dates), grains (barley, wheat), and honey, and whether it is by cooking or natural fermentation is due to its peculiarity to drink. The wine was gradually banned in the Qur'an and it was completely banned after the principle of Islamic society was established and after people realized the basis of monotheism and belief in the One God.[150] Allah is addressing the believers, that is, those to whom the faith has already been established and in their hearts and to whom these religious regulations refer.

In addition to wine, in the verse for alcohol, Allah compares mentioned the statues and arrows (horoscope, prophecies, superstitions) which are also harmful to the human mind and society itself. The wine is described as impure. It is also the work of the devil and therefore we conclude that the mission of the devil is to seduce the believers and make them dishonest and evil in their deeds.

The Messenger of God said: *"Wine is the source of disorder and the greatest sin."* Also, he said: *"Whoever believes in Allah and the Hereafter should not sit at a table where alcohol is drinking* [152] and: *"Wine is a source of filth."*[153]

The Prophet ﷺ said: *"The angel Jibril came to me*[154] *And he said to me: 'O Muhammad, Allah has cursed the wine and the one who makes it, the one who seeks it, the one who drinks it, the one who carries it, the one to whom it is brought, the one who sells it, the one to whom it is sold, the one who it pours and to whom it's poured. '"* [155]

Tariq ibn Suwaid asked the Prophet ﷺ for the wine, so the Prophet said that it is forbidden, and Tariq said to him: *"I consider it as a medicine"*, and the Prophet said: *"It's not a cure, but is a disease."*[156]

Bukhari cites a narration related to Ibn Mas'ud which states that the Prophet ﷺ said: *" Allah has not given you any cure from what is forbidden to you."* It is also narrated that the Messenger ﷺ said: *" My ummah will indeed drink wine and name it with different names."* The Prophet said: *"Wine is everything that intoxicates the human mind."*

The Bible forbids the consumption of alcohol with the following verses: *"Wine is a mockery, brandy is a rebel; and everyone subject to them is not reasonable."* [157] *"Do not get drunk with wine! "It can only destroy you."* [158]

Drunkenness is never a pleasant experience and is often the reason people do things they would never do while sober. But scientists say that alcohol is not only not encouraged to behave inadequately, but it also causes you to be shameless. Researchers from the University of Missouri claim that drunk people are aware when they make a mistake, but their alcohol reduces the signals to their brain that would tell them to worry about such behavior.

Alcohol helps us to make more mistakes. When we make mistakes, the activity in the area of the brain responsible for monitoring behavior increases. It sends a signal to other areas of the brain to tell them that something is wrong. "Our research has shown that alcohol does not reduce the ability of people to know I made a mistake but causes less to worry about making those mistakes, "- said prof. Bruce Bartholomew, who led the study. To reach this conclusion, prof. Bartholomew and his colleagues monitored the brain activity of young people aged 21 to 35 years. One-third of the participants were given an alcoholic beverage, and the rest were not given alcohol or they used a placebo drink. Then, everyone had to perform a certain task on the computer. The results showed that participants who drank alcohol were aware of making a mistake, but simply did not care. Even after the mistake was made, the drunken participants did not slow down to become more careful, as the sober ones do.

As it is known, in the USA, it is allowed to drive with 0.08% blood alcohol. However, new research from the University of California shows that driving with even a small amount of alcohol is not safe.[159]

On the other hand, the French, and then the rest of the world, got to their feet with the news of the alleged decades-long delusion about the healing properties of wine. According to some new research, "a glass a day" increases the risk of cancer.[160]

Therefore, the statement of Muhammad should not be surprising: *"Alcohol is the mother of all evils."*[161]

Transmitted by Ummu Selema: *"The Prophet forbade everything that intoxicates and causes weakness (mufetir)."*

Mufetir is all that causes apathy, and apathy is insensitivity, weakness, stimulated relaxation of the body, and unresponsive to external factors, and without a doubt, all this is caused by drugs and narcotics.

The harmfulness of cigarette smoking

Tell me which of you would put rat poison in the food you love the most? Would you poison yourself? So how can smokers smoke knowing that one cigarette contains as much as one rat poison and more ?!This, of course, includes alcoholic beverages, but also narcotics.

A report by the US Department of Health says that the number of victims of smoking in the USA has reached about 360,000 people a year and fifty thousand as victims of secondhand smoke.

In Britain, that number is over 100,000 smokers a year. The report of the World Health Organization states that the number of those who die or live an unhealthy life caused by smoking undoubtedly exceeds the number of those who die from the plague, cholera, measles, typhoid, and the like.

It is noticeable that more and more Americans are quitting smoking, but on the other hand more and more believers and people in whose traditions smoking was not widespread, it is used more and more.

If you are a smoker and have a heart problem, the best and most effective way to protect your heart from stroke is to quit smoking. Smoking not only leads to heart failure but also causes lung cancer, pancreatic cancer, and can lead to stroke, chronic bronchitis, and more. Sick person becomes a burden to the family and its treatment is quite complicated and difficult. Smoking is also associated with impotence in men and infertility in women.

The benefits of quitting smoking are noticeable from the first day you quit smoking. And within five years of quitting smoking, depending on the person, the chance of developing coronary artery disease in the heart is similar to those who did not smoke at all. A great number of Islamic scholars issued fatwas[162] for banning smoking due to the great harm it causes. Whoever wants to get rid of smoking and tobacco will have to act strongly, firmly, and decisively. This requires strong faith and conviction in the safety of smoking. Every believer should make a mental picture how he will appear in front of his Lord on the Day of Judgment when he will be asked how he treated his body and life given to him by the Creator.

The 1994 medical book *Current* tells us about some of the benefits of quitting smoking:

- Improves breathing power;
- The sense of smell and taste returns;
- You need less time to fall asleep;
- Improves physical strength;
- The danger of passive smoking to other people is reduced;
- Improves the vitality of arteries and veins;
- The heart rate decreases;
- The money will be saved and the possibility of making a fire etc. will be reduced.

The harm of marijuana to human health

The Prophet Muhammad ﷺ said: *"Everything which intoxicates is haram."*[163]

Many clinical studies have examined the harmful effects of cannabis on human health. Marijuana Damages Human DNA Molecule According to researchers, there is strong evidence that cannabis smoke damages human DNA molecules. This damage to the DNA molecule also increases the risk of cancer. Scientists in the UK have discovered, in laboratory conditions, that cannabis smoke damages the DNA molecule. They published their research in *Chemical Research in Toxicology*.

There are many studies on the toxicity of cigarette smoke. Cigarette smoke is known to contain 4,000 chemicals, 60 of which are carcinogenic. In contrast, cannabis has not been well researched. Cannabis smoke (marijuana) contains 400 chemicals, including cannabinoids. But cannabis smoke contains 50% more carcinogenic polycyclic aromatic hydrocarbons, such as naphthalene, benzanthracene, and benzopyrene, than cigarette smoke, if it transmits others.

As reports the English magazine "*The Independent* ", high rate of testicular cancer in the UK, as well as in other Western countries, today is linked to the growing consumption of cannabis. The incidence of testicular cancer has more than doubled in the last 30 years, which is attributed to the increasing consumption of this, by far the most popular illegal drug in the UK. Scientists have found that men who smoke cannabis regularly have a 70% higher risk of developing testicular cancer than men who have never smoked cannabis in their lives. The risk is twice as high in men who have smoked cannabis at least once a week or have been smokers for a long time, starting in their teens, than in those who have never used the drug.[164]

A recent study found that marijuana also causes memory loss in laboratory mice. The scientists add that this knowledge could be of great help in researching cannabis and its use for medical purposes. Cannabis has long been known to cause memory loss because it has a direct effect on the part of the brain that manages cognitive functions, according to *Nature Neuroscience* magazine.

But does forgetfulness last only during consumption or does consumption have long-term consequences? - These are questions that scientists are still debating. What is important is that the person who consumes marijuana acquires a completely different consciousness, with lethargy, and is not interested in the phenomena around him, which indirectly harms himself and those with whom he lives. A separate chapter should be devoted to marijuana and narcotics, but the harmfulness of this substance and its long-term consequences are visible in society.

Overeating

The Messenger of God, warns us of the danger of overeating and belching that occurs as a result. Ibn Umar r.a. says: *"Someone in the company of the Messenger of God supported him so he said:"Listen, spare us from your belching, because those who were the least hungry in this world, will be the hungriest one in the afterlife."*[165]

In the Musnad it is noted that the Prophet ﷺ said: *"Man has not filled a worse tank than his stomach. Therefore, it will be enough for the sons of Adam to satisfy their hunger with a few bites to regain their strength. "If he has to eat, then he should reserve one-third of his stomach for food, one-third for water, and one-third for normal breathing."*

Overeating leads to indigestion, which can lead to insomnia. Scientist Pierre Flocher says: "A third of humanity die because there is not enough food and drink. The second third of people die from eating too much."

Therefore, there are two types of diseases, it is heart disease and physical disease that is a consequence of the entry of ingredients whose action impairs the natural functions and balance of the body, and this is the type of general disease that affects most people. This disease is most often caused by overeating, taking food before the previous food is digested, eating tough food that is slow to digest, eating foods with a deficient composition, eating and mixing foods with opposite flavors, or specially prepared sweets for the same meal. When the body gets used to this type of unhealthy diet, it will inherit various types of diseases. That is why we say that moderation is the path to good health, and the body is used in moderation and the diet should be moderate. This is because a full stomach damages the body, heart, and soul. This situation is even more difficult when it becomes a habit because the person will feel depression, sluggishness, and difficulty for both body and soul. That will neglect obedience to fundamental religious duties.[166]

Why is it forbidden to blow in hot meal?

From Abdullah Ibn Abbas was narrated that: " *Allah's Messenger forbade breathing over or blowing into the vessel.* "[167] This is a common, everyday habit of many, especially children, and we know that the Prophet ﷺ forbade this act, and he said nothing for no reason. Scientific fact says that in our bodies are located "friendly" bacteria, which unlike the harmful bacteria, helps our body to defend itself from certain diseases, and is located in the throat. However, when a person starts to blow, this bacterium comes with air from the oral cavity, and when it comes in contact with hot surfaces, it turns into harmful bacteria that leads to the appearance of cancerous cells that cause a row, God save us! Due to the foregoing advised we do not blow the hot food and drinks to be cooled.

The harm of drinking blood

Say, *"I do not find within that which was revealed to me [anything] forbidden to one who would eat it unless it is a dead animal or blood spilled out or the flesh of swine - for indeed, it is impure - or it is [that slaughtered in] disobedience, dedicated to other than Allah. But whoever is forced [by necessity], neither desiring [it] nor transgressing [its limit], then indeed, your Lord is Forgiving and Merciful."* (Qur'an, 6:145)
The prohibition is specifically linked to the blood that *flows out* when the animal has been slaughtered on a halal way, i.e. by cutting the jugular veins and carotid arteries, and does not extend to trace amounts that remain in the flesh after being drained and washed, etc. "

Consumption of blood was a custom of the Arabs and Islam strictly forbade it. These Qur'anic verses show that the net consumption of the meat of a slaughtered, drowned, and slaughtered animal, the meat of a beast stabbed with a beast, is forbidden, because in this way the slaughtered animal is full of bacteria and is subject to decay and rot the meat becomes poisonous.
It was known in ancient times, but nowadays these medical aspects of these prohibitions are fully researched which found that in addition to bacteria and viruses in terms of the spread of disease is to blame a protein, prion, which does not have its genetic material. There is no way to detect it in an infected animal because it does not stimulate the development of antibodies and goes unidentified. It can not be destroyed by temperatures of 360 degrees, or by cooking at 130 degrees, nor can it be destroyed by radiation, which means that it is indestructible. It is the cause of various diseases, among which is the disease known as *mad cow* disease. Everyone who eats this meat substance, including

dogs, cats, and humans, became ill and die with symptoms of this terrible disease. The biggest culprit of all this is that the disease spread because the cows were fed processed food from extinct sheep which was later given to humans and this caused death in many people and unprecedented damage. Processed feathers, processed animals that have died, the processed litter of orange peel, almonds, chicken manure are given to cows that people fed on to get more milk.

 Dr. Virgill Hulse and Stephen Dealer who are professors at the University of Leeds, categorically assert and explain their scientific research. As for the blood that is in a liquid state, a healthy person refuses it and refrains from consuming it, and not to make delicious food from it. First of all, the blood itself is impure and is the cause of various diseases. The blood mixes very quickly with the dirty matter, ie with the viruses and bacteria that are in the air. Its red color decays immediately after death, after being present inside the body in a liquid state when it had certain nutritional functions. It is difficult to digest and has a detrimental effect on physical health because it ferments in the digestive tract.

That is why it is forbidden to eat a dead animal in all religions because it will cause great harm. As for the blood, it also refers to the dead animal. If a horse weighing 700 kg is injected with an injection that contains only a part of the millionth part of the blood of the killed animal, it would be irritated (rage). That is why Islam has strictly set the conditions for sacrificing animals, so that it is healthy, without diseases, and does not harm those who will consume its meat.

Horns are also a source of infection and if an animal were to transmit that infection through the horns to the organs of another animal, an epidemic and infectious disease could occur that could be transmitted to humans other than animals. That is why it is forbidden to consume food from an animal stained with horns.

The hadith narrated by Ahmed and Ibn Majah who has narrated from Abdullah ibn Umar that the Prophet said:

"You are allowed the meat of two kinds of dead animals and two kinds of blood, the flesh of a dead whale and a locust, and the blood of the liver and spleen."

This does not mean only the whale, but its meaning is broader and refers to fish in general and all seafood. The locust is mentioned because it has no blood it does not spoil and is not harmful to eat.

The blood of the liver and spleen is the only allowed blood because those two organs are formed from blood, so it is a blood clot and is not in a liquid state, and it does not produce harmful bacteria as in ordinary blood unless left for a while unprotected.

Fasting

In recent times, increasingly serious medical studies confirmed the benefits of Islamic fasting in health issues. Namely, because Muslims respect the imperative of the first Qur'anic revelation: *Iqre,* that is, read or learn. Serious scientific papers appear that reveal the benefits of Ramadan fasting for human health. Because the benefits of fasting are so numerous, it is often referred to as "operation without a knife".

One of the scientifically established ways is Intermittent fast, additionally referred to as intermittent energy restriction. It's an umbrella term for varied meal temporal order schedules that cycle between voluntary fasting (or reduced calorie intake) and non-fasting over a given period. Three ways of intermittent fast are alternate-day fast, periodic fast, and daily time-restricted feeding. Intermittent fast is also similar to a calorie-restriction diet,[2] and has been studied within the twenty first century as a practice to probably scale back the danger of diet-related diseases, like metabolic syndrome.

The science concerning intermittent fasting is contested. The American Heart Association (AHA) states that intermittent fasting[8] may produce weight loss, reduce insulin resistance, and lower the risk of cardiometabolic diseases, although its long-term sustainability is unknown. The US National Institute on Aging states that there is insufficient evidence to recommend intermittent fasting and encourages speaking to one's healthcare provider about the benefits and risks before making any significant changes to one's eating pattern. But, a 2019 review concluded that intermittent fasting may help with obesity, insulin resistance, dyslipidemia, hypertension, and inflammation.[9]

The scientific journal *Annals of Nutrition and Metabolism has* published several scientific papers on the impact of fasting on human health. We will summarize some of those papers.[170] When the body does not receive food, it begins to burn fat for more energy. It can lead to weight loss. However, if you fast for too long, your body will start using muscle protein as an energy source, which is not healthy.

Dr.Razeen Mahran is anesthetist from Oxford, she says there is a strong link between diet and health. "We should not think of Ramadan as an opportunity to lose weight, because the spiritual aspect is more important than the

---

[8] https://en.wikipedia.org/wiki/Intermittent_fasting
[9] de Cabo, Rafael; Mattson, Mark P. (December 2019). "Effects of intermittent fasting on health, aging, and disease". *New England Journal of Medicine*. **381** (26): 2541–51. doi:10.1056/NEJMra1905136

health aspect," he said. However, Ramadan is a great opportunity to improve the condition of our bodies. The changes that occur in the body during fasting depend on the duration of the fast. The body enters a state of fasting eight hours after the last meal when the absorption of nutrients from food ends in the intestines. A normal main source of energy is glucose stored in the liver and muscles. During fasting, these glucose accumulation are first used as an energy source. Later, when glucose is depleted, the body begins to consume the same fats as an energy source. Small amounts of energy are also produced in other processes in the liver. If fasting lasts for days or weeks, the body will begin to use protein as an energy source.

This is a technical description of what is otherwise known as "starvation". It involves the release of protein from the muscles, so from here the hungry people look very lean and weak. However, during Ramadan, there is unlikely to be a phase of starvation, as fasting is broken every day.

Since Ramadan fasting lasts only from sunrise to sunset, the power supply can be compensated with iftar(first meal after fasting) and sifir (last meal before fasting).

This gradually shifts from the use of glucose to the use of fat as the main source of energy and prevents the destruction of protein in muscle. Dr.Mahran said that using fat as an energy source helps to reduce weight, protects muscles, and reduces cholesterol levels. Weight loss will be followed by fatigue and constant tiredness. "It comes to detoxification because all the toxins that are found in fat are shattered and thrown the body." - said Dr. Mahran.

After a few days of fasting, the level of certain hormones (endorphins) in the blood increases, which makes us awake and gives a feeling of mental health.

A balanced diet and fluid intake between the two minute periods of fasting is very important. The kidneys are very effective in retaining water and salts, such as sodium and potassium, in the body. To prevent muscle wasting, meals must be made up of foods that are high in energy sources, such as carbohydrates and some fats.

Austrian doctor, 80 – year old, R.Broyce claims in his book: *Cancer, leukemia, and other seemingly incurable diseases treatable naturally*, that cancer can be cured with the help of fasting by internal forces that every organism has.

However, we have very little respect for that inner strength. Bryce's method of treatment with fasting is based on the theory that during fasting, to maintain the body's vital organs, the body must "eat the tumor and everything that does not belong to the body."

One who is familiar with fasting immediately understands the essence, because during fasting the body gets rid of everything that does not belong to it, so in reality, the body separates what is sick from healthy, as long as the body has own reserves of strength and the patient has hope in the belief in the existence of divine healing forces within himself. This inner strength is worth trying.

Bryce often recalls that tumor outgrowth is independent and that may disappear solely by fasting because incurred in the wrong diet. We know from experience that when the body renounces food, it gets rid of everything foreign to it, i.e. of everything that does not belong to the organism.

The role of fasting in the treatment of mental illness

It does not take much knowledge to know the value of Islamic fasting for human health. Today, not only scientific magazines and professional medical books write about it, but also those who are not in the least inclined towards the faith.

Psychotherapy means healing of the soul. It is little known that psychiatry also attaches great importance to fasting. Scientifically speaking, it is a method of treatment that is applied to all neuroses, and in some cases to psychosis. Worth noting are the results obtained by the Russian psychiatrist Dr. J. Nikolaev, a doctor at a mental health clinic not far from Moscow. He successfully applied the new procedure in the treatment of the mentally ill, a therapy that consists of a complete and long fast. Food refusal is a common syndrome of acute schizophrenia. Until now, such patients have been forcibly fed. However, Dr. Nikolaev understood such a reaction as a spontaneous rejection of the food of the sick organism, so he came up with the idea to try to apply methods of total fasting. During the fast, the sick received only water, vitamin injections, and some mineral salts. The Discovery of Dr. Nikolaev is important on the other hand. This, in turn, supports one of the most recent and significant hypotheses about the onset of schizophrenia. According to that hypothesis, schizophrenia is an organic disease of physiological nature caused by a metabolic disorder, ie. chemical processes in the patient's body, during which some toxic substances are created that negatively affect the work of the brain, in fact as a drug. Fasting, according to Nikolaev, allows the body to "purify" itself of those substances, to establish its metabolic balance and to heal.

Fasting heals the body and soul without any special operating expense. Fasting is a great ally of humans. [171]

Islamic psychology and its impact on health

Crying as a medicine

Crying is an emotional bond with God and a way to draw closer to Him. It should be done sincerely and the best and most beautiful tear is the tear shed in solitude towards our Creator.

Bayhaqi narrates a narration from Abu Hurairah, radiyallahu anhu, where he says: *"After the verse was revealed:* ***"Do you wonder at this speech and laugh and do not weep?"****[172], and the people of Saffa wept so much* *that tears flowed down their cheeks, after which the Prophet ﷺ, if he heard their whining and he would start crying with them and then we would cry because of his crying."*

It is also narrated that Ibn Umar r.a. in reciting the chapter al-Mutafifin, read the verse, ***"On the day when people will be raised for the sake of their Lord."***[173] so he began to weep until he lost consciousness, for which he did not complete the surah(chapter). The best tear is the tear in solitude. He who sleeps in solitude before his Lord will be one of the saved on the Day of Judgment. He will be in the group of 7 chosen in the shade of Allah's Throne. [174]

But what does science say about this? The eyes produce different tears. There are three types: Permanent or basal tears are created to retain moisture in the eyes. With each blink, the eyelids shed tears all over the eyes. Reflex tears are created as a reaction to irritation or due to the presence of a foreign body. Emotional tears are produced as a result of various emotions - sadness, pain, happiness, anger, frustration, and the like. Scientists have analyzed the composition of different tears and have concluded that emotional tears have a different composition from tears caused by irritation. Emotional tears contain enzymes, immunoglobulins, and proteins not found in other types of tears. There is an unproven theory that crying is a method to get rid of toxins produced by stress hormones, and therefore it is considered to be beneficial to health. After expressing their emotions through crying, most people feel more relaxed. Almost 90% of "crying people" feel better and are happier after shedding tears.

After crying, breathing and heart rate slow down, sweating decreases, and a period of relaxation occurs that lasts longer than the crying itself. As a result, some people remember relaxation better than crying. Research has shown that people who cry as a result of stress, pain, or other strong emotions are generally healthier than those who do not.

It is well known that emotional retention leads to increased stress levels, which can contribute to headaches, depression, heart disease, and many other ailments. It can be said that crying is one way for the body to fight stress.

So the next time you feel tears welling up in your eyes, do not be afraid to let them flow. Just let them pour for something really important. And what is more important than our happy ending in this world and seeing the joy of the afterlife?

Mentioning God brings peace

 David B. Larson,[10] of the American National Research Center for Health, and his team, compered between pious and non-religious Americans getting very surprising results. For example, religious people experience 60% less heart disease than those with little or no faith at all, when it comes to suicide then the percentage rises to almost 100% for non-religious people. Religious people have a much lower level of high pressure, and this ratio in smokers is 7: 1.

According to the results of the research, those who do not believe in God, are subject to double the suffering of

---

[10] https://spiritualityandhealth.duke.edu/index.php/scholars/david-b-larson

internal abdominal pain compared to the believers, and their mortality when it comes to respiratory diseases is even 66% higher than that of the believers. Secular psycho lineages tend to prove that it applies to the so-called "psychological effect". Yet it proves that belief in Allah is far stronger than any other psychological influence.

The large and wide range of research on the connection between religious belief and psychological well-being presented by Dr. Herbert Benson[11] of the Faculty of Medicine at Harvard produced surprising conclusions in this area of research. Even though he is not a believer, Dr. Benson concluded that worship and belief in Allah have a more positive effect on human health than any other belief. Benson told us that faith does not contribute with so much mental peace as it contributes to belief in something particular like God.

What is the reason for this connection between the belief of the human soul and the body? The conclusion reached by Benson is in his words that the human body and mind are regulated to believe in God. This fact, which the world of medicine has slowly begun is a secret revealed in the Qur'an in these words:

" Who have believed and whose hearts have rest in the remembrance of Allah. Verily in the remembrance of Allah do hearts find rest! (Qur'an, Ar-Rad, 28)

Allah is the Giver of peace, the One who is pure from all imperfections and whose characteristics are far from inconsistent. His activities are cleansed of evil and are the source of all peaceful work throughout the universe. Allah's divine deeds are free from all evil which is in itself, just as no evil on earth is without any hidden good in it. Allah is the giver of peace, saves the believer from torture, and welcomes them with a greeting of peace in a home that will

---

[11] https://bensonhenryinstitute.org/about-us-dr-herbert-benson/

last forever. Glory be to Allah, He is the Giver of Peace in this world and the Hereafter.

"... and on the Day when they will meet Him, He will greet them with: 'Peace be with you!'And He has prepared for them a noble reward."[178]

The reason that those who believe in Allah, pray and obey Him, and are mentally and physically healthy is that they act following their cause of creation. Philosophies and systems that oppose human creation and its cause of creation always lead to pain and misfortune.

Modern medicine is currently striving to realize this truth. As Patrick Glynn said: *"Scientific research in psychology over the past 25 years has shown that religious belief is one of the strongest interrelationships of overall mental health and happiness."* [179]

The great secret of faith is hidden in the fact that the heart will not achieve peace, tranquility, and stability except by establishing a relationship with his Lord. It is the love of the One. He whose love, desires, and obedience end up with someone other than Allah, indeed he will fail at the moment when he needs it most. And whoever loves, fears, hopes, and aims at Allah, the Exalted, will attain eternal grace, joy, serenity, and happiness. As much as a servant of God is committed and persistent in carrying out the provisions of the faith, he receives gentleness in determining the provisions of destiny. If he obeys all the provisions of the faith, formally and substantially, then he is given gentleness and compassion (el lutf), formally and substantially. However, if he performs the provisions of the faith formally and neglects the essence and the basis, then he is limited to the formality, while in essence, its influence is negligible...[180]

Optimism and pessimism

The beautiful word, when heard, cheers and gives optimism (hope). Muhammad, said: *"I like optimism."*[181]
Pessimism is a bad opinion of Allah, subhanahu wa ta'ala, and attributing to Him the inherent things of someone else, associating the heart with something that has been created for a day that does not use or make harm. Optimism is a good opinion of Allah that does not deter a person from his needs.
This is nowadays medically proven. Pessimistic people are at greater risk of developing heart problems than optimists. This is revealed by a study presented at the assembly of the Swedish Medical Association.
In Islam, pessimism is condemned and given no room. In every situation, even the most tragic one such as death, a way is sought to resort to positive optimism.
Analogously, the reality is confirmed by Islamic law, that victory belongs to the belief. Hence, there is no room for hopelessness and pessimism. One should try to give the maximum of each individual effort and then rely on the One who is Almighty. Whoever says that he is optimistic, and withdraws from deeds and work, he is incompetent, and not at all optimistic. It is narrated in one poem:
"A wise person is one who is self-critical towards his soul and does deeds that will benefit him after his death, and an ignorant person is one who follows the instincts of his soul and hopes for the help of Allah."
Optimism encourages man to work and remove his despair from his soul. It guides man in his effort to get over all obstacles. Such a person can overcome all difficulties, both health and psychological.

106

- "And We will surely test you with something of fear and hunger and a loss of wealth and lives, but give good tidings to the patient..." [182]

According to the knowledge of modern science, mercy comes in the form of improved health. Bernard Jansen, in his book *The Science and Practice of Iridology,* states: *"Doctors today recognize that the most important human workshop is not the physical body but the mind that controls it."* Dr. Ted Morter says the same in his book, *Your Health,* which says it is your choice to say that the bad thoughts are manufacturer of acids in the body (a high level of acidity is the reason for some diseases) because your body responds to negative mental and emotional stress that produces thoughts in the same way as it responds to "real" dangers from physical threats. Hospital examinations show that 70% of the respondents, quasi - patients, did not have an organic basis for their health complaints. In these patients, although there was no organic basis for their illness, it was caused by psychological grounds. Since Freud popularized the idea ofpsychoanalysis, people often turn to the realm of mental reality to solve certain problems, forgetting that we can not separate physical and mental reality. The mind is part of the brain, and the brain is an organ. Like all organs, it feeds on the same source of nutrients as other organs that are prone to the same problems. After all, the brain is just a part of our body as any other part and is completely dependent on the body. It needs sugar to produce energy, unlike other organs that produce it from potassium and fat. Therefore, the brain is the first organ that responds to a lack of sugar and reacts most sharply. Freud stated that psychoanalysis was not suitable for the treatment of diseases such as schizophrenia and pointed out that its causes were biochemical. The brain uses the same bloodstream where we can understand how the brain can physically affect us. For example, by simply using our brains to think and learn, we burn nutrients in our

107

system, especially phosphorus. Heavy stress on the brain can cause a lack of phosphorus, so people with high IQs need high levels of phosphorus. Phosphorus is not the only nutritious thing that can be consumed under psychological stress and with little spiritual calm. If the thyroid gland, the organ that controls our senses, works overtime, iodine deficiency can occur.

Very great wisdom lies in the narration transmitted by Muhammad ﷺ: *"It is not strong, the one who defeats people with his strength, but the one who controls himself in anger. "*[183] Restraint in peace and patience is the key to physical strength. Stress from work, divorce, or death can cause a loss of potassium and sodium in the body because it causes the thyroid gland to have an increased need for this mineral. Even hypoglycemia (high blood sugar) can be caused by arousal. The Prophet ﷺ recommended a moderate path in life. However, we often get into or get exposed to intense physiological condition by shouting, watching too much television, and going to places of entertainment, and often in those situations the adrenal cortex is stimulated and blood sugar rises. This in turn stimulates the pancreas causing fatigue or weakness. Comfortable and health wearable pretext is doing thing with exposing gratitude to Allah - saying *alhamdulillah*, especially when we have a problem. We should try to keep the home and work environment calm, without stressful situations as much as possible. One of the ways we can reduce the effects of stress is to be aware of stress itself, to eat nutrients and supplements such as herbs and the like. If a person performs ibadah [acts of worship of the Almighty God] late at night or reads the Qur'an during Ramadan, he must eat foods rich in phosphorus and one that will help maintain strength due to concentration. If we travel or perform Hajj, we need the intake of foods rich in potassium, sodium and vitamin B complex. The quantity must be increased due to physical exertion and muscle strain. In most health problems, prevention itself is far superior to finding a cure.

Therefore, the best way to avoid negative attitudes and emotions to take control of our bodies is to practice the wisdom that Allah has given us in the Qur'an and the hadiths. We should say alhamdulillah (praise be to Allah) about what we have, inshaAllah (if Allah wills) what we intend, and Subhanallah (praise be to Allah) when we see something exciting and wonderful. Astaghfirullah (may Allah forgive) we should say when we get upset or weak and most importantly Allahu Akbar (Allah is Great) when we face the challenges of life. These five expressions regularly mentioned are like a multivitamin for our complete health. I ask Allaah to provide me and you with positive optimism that creates deeds that will remove us from our idleness and weakness.

Morning and night prayer as a remedy

The book *"Home Recipes and Secrets of Natural Healing"*, written in English by a group of authors in 1993, states: *"Getting out of bed and moving around the house, as well as doing lighter physical exercises, as well as rubbing hands and feet with water and taking deep breaths have many health benefits. "*

Anyone who thinks about these tips will find that they completely agree with taking ablution and praying when getting up for a night for prayer. Messenger indicates the value of the performance of the night prayer, and said: *"Perform the night prayer, because it is a characteristic of the good people in front of you, a nice way of approaching*

How does night prayer remove diseases from the body? Namely, modern science has confirmed the following: "Getting up overnight reduces the secretion of the hormone cortisol, and especially before waking up from sleep for several hours, which coincides with the period before dawn (the last third of the night). This prevents a sudden rise in blood sugar, which is a special danger for diabetics. Also, this hormone is the cause of a sharp rise in blood pressure, which leads to stroke and heart disease, especially in patients who already feel these symptoms.

Also, the night prayer reduces the possibility of blood clotting in the veins of the sensory receptor networks that occur due to the slow flow of blood during sleep. This reduces the chance of blood thrombosis due to low fluid intake or dehydration or obesity and shortness of breath, which makes it difficult for blood to return to the head.

The night and morning prayers bring improvement to the patients with arthritis, be it rheumatism or any other similar disease, which occurs as a result of movement and rubbing with water while taking ablution.

Night prayer is a successful cure for what is called 'chronic fatigue' as a reason for aligning the movements in the form of lower and moderate exertion, which has shown its results in the treatment of this disease.

Night and morning prayers improve the reduction of triglycerides (a type of fat) that accumulate in the blood, which exposes a person to the danger of vascular disease. These fats are in 32% of cases the cause of vascular disease. Night and morning prayer reduces the risk of death in all circumstances, and especially a death that may be of myocardial consequential stroke, and certain types of tumors. Also, the night prayer reduces the risk of sudden death due to impaired heart function. Getting up early is an occasion to breathe the morning air that we know is clean of contamination during the day.

The night and morning prayers activate the human memory as well as the various intellectual functions of the brain because in the night prayers the Qur'an is learned and pondered, prayers are recited and zikr is repeated. Night and morning prayers are a reason to protect ourselves from Alzheimer's disease, senility, depression, and others. Also, the night prayer reduces and prevents the disease of tinnitus which occurs more often for unknown reasons.

Experts from the Jordanian Association of Cardiologists have confirmed that performing the morning prayer at its scheduled time each day is the best way to prevent and treat heart disease and atherosclerosis, as well as myocardial infarction and vascular disease. can be the cause of a stroke. This confirmation came as a result of modern scientific study on heart disease and atherosclerosis that made this association in Jordan. The medical research confirmed that the diseased from the myocardium of the heart is in danger situation, and the main reason for atherosclerosis disease and clothing of blood vessels is a late-night sleep or during the day. The Prophet Muhammad said: *"The blessing of this ummah(Islamic nation) is in the early awakening"*[186]

The results of these studies confirmed the above hadith which confirmed our knowledge of what a great blessing is human health. These studies have exposed that when a person sleeps for a long time, the heart rate decreases and they do not exceed fifty per minute. When the heart rate decreases, the blood flows far more slowly through the blood vessels, which leads to the deposition of salts and fats on the walls of the blood vessels, especially those that carry blood to and from the heart. A heart attack then occurs, or the arteries that carry blood to the brain become completely blocked, leading to a stroke, which in most cases is fatal.

The results of these studies particularly emphasized the obligation to abstain from prolonged sleep, so that one sequence of sleep should not last more than four hours - when it is necessary to get up and perform an activity lasting at least fifteen minutes, which we find it daily in the performance of the morning prayer in the first hours of the dawn. The prayer is best performed in a mosque, which also means physical activity in early morning hours.

.

The scientific aspect of prostration

Electromagnetic waves perform radiation through different electronic devices that we use daily, such as TV, objects of remote, mobile phones, computers, and so on. We are one of those who receive large amounts of electromagnetic waves. In other words, we are charged with electromagnetic waves, and we do not even notice it!

We have headaches! We feel uncomfortable! Laziness at work and pain in different parts of the body! Do not forget this when you experience some of these symptoms. What is the solution to all this?

Scientist and cardiologist, Dr. Stephan Sinatra conducted a study that concluded that the best way for the body to remove these harmful electromagnetic waves that injure the body is a process called grounding. Dr. Ibrahim Kazim confirms this and says: *"more frequent lowering of the forehead to the ground so that the earth absorbs the harmful electromagnetic waves"*. [187]

This is similar to a building, where an electrical signal (such as thunder) will be absorbed through the ground. That is why we need to lower our foreheads to the ground to remove these harmful electromagnetic signals. What makes this research strange is that it is best to lower our heads to the sand or the ground.

According to Dr. Ibrahim, the best way to lower our foreheads is while we are in a position facing the geographical center of the Earth. In this way, we will remove the electromagnetic signals better and more efficiently. It is interesting to note that Mecca is the geographical center of the world and Kaba is located exactly at the geographical center of the Earth.

With that the prostration[188] In our prayers, it is the best way to rid ourselves of electromagnetic field from our body. It is also the best way to be closer to Allah, subhanahu wa ta'ala, Who created this universe in such a original way. Almighty Allah always asks us to do things that help us and that are useful to us. There are cases when we do not know the reason for a prescribed religious act, but sooner or later we find the reason. In any case, we must believe in Almighty Allah and we must know that whatever we do for Him, it is best for us! Finally, we do not prostrate to remove this electromagnetic energy, but to obey Almighty Allah. We believe that there is always mercy and great wisdom in His commands.

There is always scientific evidence for every command, and it is important to show people that whatever Muslims do and it is recommended by the Qur'an and the hadiths is good for them![189]

Impact of odors on human health

Muhammad ﷺ said: " *Among the things of this world, women are most dear to me and fragrances, and the freshness of my eye (the joy of my heart) is in prayer.* " [190]

Lately, it has been scientifically proven that scents have a major impact on the body and psyche of man. Thus, the smell of lavender does make you drowsy, the smell of cinnamon makes us creative, rose and vanilla makes us courageous. Aromatic plant extracts (essential oils) have been used for medicinal purposes for centuries, even today. Thus, while lavender relaxes and calms, eucalyptus clears the mind and gives energy. Mind-boggling, but it is true that by inhaling natural aromatic oil we can get rid of and significantly alleviate negative emotions, stress, fear, anger, sadness, depression, pain, and at the same time encourage positive emotions such as joy, pleasure.

 Professor Boris Stack and co-workers at Mannheim Hospital analyzed the effect of smells on the emotions that arise during sleep. Thus, those respondents who were exposed to the scent of roses after waking up said that they felt positive emotions, while the group that was exposed to the stench of rotten eggs reported a completely different effect.

Aromatherapy is an ancient skill of applying essential oils in various ways for relaxation, prevention, and treatment. It dates back to ancient civilizations. Essential oils are obtained by distillation, a process that was invented 2500 years ago. People then found how to take the essence-soul and the smell from the plants. The distillation process is quite simple. The plants (leaves, twigs, roots, resin) are closed in a container under which a fire is lit. By heating the vessel, steam is created which will take with it both the active compounds and the odors in the cooling pipes. They condense and turn the steam into a mixture of water and essential oils that float on its surface. Thus, on one side the water is separated, and on the other the essential oil. Getting a few drops of essential oil requires a large amount of plant material.

The ancient civilizations knew that it was the essence of plants and they knew how to appreciate those few drops.

As they are strong concentrates of plants, they should be applied very carefully. They are not used as concentrated oils but are diluted with other neutral oils such as almond and others. Otherwise, they can lead to side effects such as burns, allergic reactions, nausea, dizziness, and even poisoning.

Oils with their ability to regenerate tissues can increase the body's reduced resistance. With the help of aromatherapy methods, the essential oils quickly penetrate the bloodstream, through which they are distributed to all parts of the body. They restore harmony and have a beneficial effect on organs and systems whose functional balance is disturbed. There is no essential oil that works on just one disease or one type of ailment. The best example of this is lavender oil, which in addition to being an antiseptic, also works to reduce fatigue and depression, improve mood, and thus work to reduce chronic pain.

Inhalation of aromatic oils can alleviate fear, anxiety, tension, stress, pain, improve memory, and concentration. Although we usually rely on what we see and hear, smells play an important role in our lives.

Impact of colors on human health

The word green is mentioned many times in the Qur'an when describing the condition of the people of Paradise and what surrounds them: prosperity and luxury, happiness, and contentment. For example, Allah, subhanahu wa ta'ala, says in the Qur'an:

"They will be leaning on green seats, covered with rugs, magical and beautiful ..."[191]

What do psychologists say? Dr. Ardtcham[192] found that colors have a certain effect on humans. To prove this claim, he conducted several experiments that show how color affects our mood, our sense of warmth and cold, our happiness or sorrow, and our personality and the way we view life. Today, hospitals pay attention to the role that colors play when it comes to the interior of the person and seek expert opinion on what color should be the walls and clothes of staff.

Experiments have shown that yellow stimulates the nervous system. Orange brings security and calm, blue makes people feel cold, unlike red which makes them feel warm. However, it turns out that the color of joy and happiness is green and that makes it a favorite color for operating rooms and uniforms. Here we will mention an experiment that was conducted in London, on the London bridge, the place which was known for the numerous suicides committed on it. After its gray color was changed to a beautiful green color, the number of suicides was significantly reduced. It is also known that the green color facilitates the view due to the small area ofvisibility along the middle wavelength which is shorter than the red one and longer than the blue one.[193]

Excessive emotions cause diseases

Emotions are an indispensable everyday element in human life. Ordinary human emotions have a great influence on the organs, ie on their functioning and health.

Joy is a feeling of deep satisfaction, and it is connected with the heart. When we are very excited, due to great joy we can feel some negative symptoms such as anxiety, insomnia, fever, and a strong heartbeat. True joy is not experienced in this world and therefore the believer should give thanks to Allah when he rejoices in something.

Anger is an emotion that is associated with insults, frustrations, nervousness, and anger. This mood reflects on the liver and digestive fluid. Anger drains energy and causes headaches, dizziness, and raises blood pressure. The believer should, therefore, before getting angry, take a deep breath, dedicate your thoughts to the Creator and say: ***We are all from God, and to Him, we all return.*** The Prophet said: *"Patience is at the first strike,"* because believer was allowed to fall into a state of mental incompetence and lay unrest and fear, and in these times know the real heroes who are patient in the most difficult moments.

Anxiety is an emotion that is the result of excessive anxiety and can affect the lungs and intestines. People can not use the energy they have because of the feeling of restlessness, they suffer from shortness of breath, ulcers, and inflammatory processes in the intestines. The unrest of this world will not disappear unless you, as a believer, have secured the best deal, and that is to use this world in the worship of the Creator so the unrest will completely disappear in the other world .

Sadness does not encourage just tears but creates disharmonic lungs. Grief can take away our willpower, damage our lungs, and cause respiratory illness.

Melancholy affects bad temper, resulting in fatigue, lethargy, and poor concentration. Some scientific studies claim that it can also affect the digestive organs and cause bloating. This feeling of emptiness the believer can change through prayer and look for new ways and methods that will fulfill him to succeed as a believer in this world and deserve the promised reward.

Fear can interfere with kidney function and is known to cause spontaneous urination. Extreme fear "shocks" the kidneys and bladder. Allah says that the fear of people is nothing in this world and that there will come a time when the ***fear will be hardened***,[194] This will be felt by every unbeliever, while the believers are promised bliss and joy.

[195] *Shock* is a state of real fear, ie *panic*. Short-term shock affects the heart, and if it lasts longer it damages the kidneys.

Because of this: *Be grateful.* Do not roll your eyes at anything that annoys you. Write down on paper the things you need to be gentle on. And that's a activity, but that way you will be reminded of the good things in your life.

Get out. Live in a large room with a high blue ceiling, fresh air, and grass floor. Just five minutes' walk outside has an effective effect on the feeling of happiness.

Have breakfast. You will not be lazy and you will cope with the tasks more easily.

Regular meals. Eat something every three to four hours and provide your body with enough energy and keep your sugar under control.

Smart time to go to bed. The body needs at least a few hours of rest to be ready for the next day. Remember that and the next time you go to bed next time.

Happy face. Countless studies have shown how a simple trick, such as a smiling face, will help you feel happier.

Put on a smile and feel better. Muhammad ﷺ told us: " *Even a smile to a brother in faith is a good deed."*[196]

Fighting stress and anger

Life is full of stress and each of us is exposed to some kind of stress. Psychological pressure is not bad in itself, but it is the way we deal with those pressures. People are not equally resistant to those pressures and some of them adapt and willingly face problems. Some of them feel an aversion to that situation, and some surrender and adapt to new circumstances. Those who experience severe crises usually have pain in the head area and the muscles of the neck and back. Some complaints of diarrhea, dizziness, and the like. Ibn Abbas r.a. was asked about anger and sadness and how does it harm the body. He said: *"They both follow the same path, but their meaning is different. When you struggle with something stronger than you, it scares you and creates sadness. And when you struggle with something weaker than you, it makes you angry."* And indeed, both feelings raise the adrenaline in the blood, raise the blood pressure, and are harmful to the heart. Some people get angry with difficulties and crises. *The Messenger of God* ﷺ *describes anger as a flame burning in the heart: "Anger is a flame burning in the heart!"*[197]

The Messenger of God ﷺ encouraged a reduction in anger:

"Whoever overcomes anger when he can retaliate, Allah will fill his heart with security and faith."

Allah tells believers that it is a virtue to forgive when the other side is in the wrong: ***"Those who give in times of both ease and hardship, those who control their rage and pardon other people — Allah loves the good-doers."*** (Qur'an, 3:134)

[198]

The Messenger of God, may Allah bless him and grant him peace, described the anger cure and said: *"If any of you get angry, let him sit down, and if the anger does not leave him, let him lie down."* (Abu Dawood, Ahmed)

Psychologists in modern times call this a change in "body condition" and believe that this change leads to a weakening of the reaction and quenching of anger. Science has found that adrenaline levels drop when you sit or lie down.

Prophet a.s. said: *"Anger is from the devil. Satan is of fire. It is extinguished with water. Whoever is angry, let him perform ablution."* There is no doubt that all these methods help, but the strongest of all methods is the belief in Allah subhanahu wa ta'ala, seeking help only from Him, patience in difficulties and patience in managing the problems. The Prophet ﷺ warned about the danger of accumulating worries: *"He who has full worries will have a sick body."* (Ahmed) Ibn Abbas narrates hadith from the Prophet ﷺthat he said: *"Whoever constantly commits istigfar (seeks forgiveness) Allah will remove all his worries, give him a way out of every situation and provide him with where he does not hope."* (Ibn Sunni Abu Nuaym)

The benefits of sleep in the fight against stress

The noble Qur'an pointed out to us the importance of sleep which gives rest to the body. Without sleep, the life of living beings could not survive on Earth. Have you ever imagined what would happen if you did not sleep? Indeed, then life would be very uncomfortable, the difficulty would prevail, there would be impaired function, overworked parts of the body to the point of destruction, weakened memory, reduced physical immunity and various diseases would appear, people would get tired and would not have rest, body cells would age and die rapidly.

Normally, long sleep is no less dangerous than insufficient sleep. Allah, the Exalted, said: ***"And We have made your dream a rest."***[199], *subat* (dream) in linguistic terminology means rest. Also, Allah, the Exalted, said in the Muhsin Khan translation of the meaning of the other verse: ***"And it is He Who makes the night a covering for you, and the sleep (as) repose, and makes the day Nushur (i.e. getting up and going for daily work, etc. after one's*** *sleep at night or like resurrection after one's death)."* (Qur'an 25:47) [200]

This is a miracle which the Qur'an pointed us in the translation of the meaning of the Qur'anic verse: *"And among His Signs is the sleep that you take by night and by day, and your seeking of His Bounty. Verily, in that are indeed signs for a people who listen."* (Qur'an 30:23) [201]

There is a saying that it is not wise to go to bed angry because the anger will accumulate even more. One research where 100 respondents took part, indicated circumstances that evoked various feelings - negative, positive and nonpartisan, and afterward, their mind motion was estimated during the REM period of rest. It was discovered that in the respondents who remained conscious for quite a while in the wake of watching the upsetting scenes, reviewing similar circumstances the following morning didn't cause an equivalent response, however, it was reduced. Then again, the respondents who headed to sleep after watching the upsetting scenes, had a similarly solid response to those scenes the following morning. It appears to be that the fantasy keeps up the enthusiastic response until the following morning. The creators of the examination noticed that numerous individuals experience difficulty dozing after an awful accident, so they presumed that it is one of the defensive systems of the mind with which sleep deprivation attempts to forestall the incitement of those feelings in memory. The best over-burden originates from destructive indignation called envy.

An Arabic proverb says, *" Never sleep with hatred for another human being."* [202] The believer should have a wide vision and subtle feelings so that he should look at things from general interest, and not through the prism of his pleasures and his ego. It is a syndrome that does not give peace. Another suggestion for better sleep is to lie down in the right way. You can lie on your back, stomach, and left or right side. Which of these positions is best for the functioning of the organism?

Dr. Atar says that a person who lies on his stomach will soon start breathing faster because the weight is on the spine and leaning on the chest will make it difficult for the chest to move, as well as their relaxation during inhalation and exhalation. Also, this lying position has the effect of bending the cervical vertebrae. What's more, it obstructs the brain respiration and heart fatigue. An Australian researcher has found that babies are more likely to die suddenly when a pregnant woman sleeps on her stomach than when she sleeps on her side. It is indisputable that these modern studies agree with what Abu Hurairah, r.a., conveys from the Prophet ﷺ : *"The Messenger saw a man lying on his stomach and said: Allah and His Messenger do not like this way of lying down."*[203]

Muhammad in the hadith recommends a short afternoon rest in the form of a dream called *kaylula*: *"Practice a short afternoon nap because the devils do not practice it!"*[204]

The saying "everything in its time" is grounded, at least when it comes to daily responsibilities and the way the human body functions.

Our metabolism follows the daily rhythm of responsibilities, so do not neglect it. Afternoon nap reduces heart disease mortality by a third as you adjust to rising levels of the sleep hormone melatonin. Just 20 minutes are enough to refresh yourself and get the energy to continue the day.

Studies have shown that afternoon nap restores energy and improves memory. If you have a chance, close your eyes briefly, but only for 30 minutes, otherwise you will wake up without energy. An afternoon nap is very healthy for the body.

Sociological aspects of impact on human health

Danger of loneliness

The Prophet Muhammad ﷺ said, *"Hold to the community, for the wolf eats the sheep which is separated from the flock."* [205]
Loneliness paves the way for a lot of bad habits, such as an unhealthy diet and lack of physical activity, thereby leading to even greater loneliness and isolation, which eventually leads to serious health problems such as a significant weakening of the immune system. It can also lead to hardening of the blood vessels, which in turn causes high blood pressure, various inflammations, and even affects the ability to remember and learn.

Loneliness causes increased secretion of the stress hormone - cortisol and dangerously increases blood pressure, which increases the chances of heart attack and stroke. Social isolation disrupts circulation and burdens the heart, and affects the quality of sleep. Scientists who have studied the impact of loneliness on health have pointed out the need to recognize the symptoms as early as possible to avoid falling into that vicious circle.

Lonely people value their social skills and interactions as less negative than they are leading to further isolation. Everyone needs some time for themselves, but if you are lonely for more than 6 months (which is considered an adjustment period if you have changed your place of residence, lost a loved one, changed jobs, etc.) you should immediately change your behavior and attitudes. You need to work on creating a positive view of the world around you and increase social physical activity, go to aerobics, play sports, take various courses, and even a walk in the park can cheer you up.

Charity cures stress

"None of you will be a true believer until he loves for his brother what he loves for himself."[206]

Prophet Muhammad ﷺ recommends helping others and meeting their needs. There are many hadiths narrated by the Prophet of Mercy, which indicate the importance of cooperating, helping others, and meeting their needs. The Noble Prophet ﷺ points out that faith is incomplete until someone begins to love his brother and what he loves for himself! He ﷺ told us that the faith of the one who sleeps comfortable is not complete if he knows that his neighbor is hungry. Whoever helps his brother in distress, Allah will help him in his distress. Whoever removes a believer's problem, Allah will remove one of his problems on the Day of Judgment. And whoever conceals a believer, Allah will conceal him on the Day of Resurrection. Based on these instructions, you notice the significance of the Prophet ﷺ care for helping others and benevolent love for them, no matter what work they have done to remove the problem from a believer in this world, to cover his shortcomings or to fulfill his need. The Noble Prophet said: *"Whoever believes in Allah and the Day of Judgment should not harm his neighbor, whoever beliefs in Allah and the Day of Judgment should honor his guest, and whoever beliefs in Allah and the Day of Judgment should say what is good or stay silent. "*[207]

Being generous to the guest is a practice that Allah (SWT) and His Messenger love and there is a great reward for it. Islam not only commands the help of others but seeks to stop and avoid insulting and harming them.

Experts in psychology confirm that helping others leads to a reduction in stress, where involvement in helping others stimulates the secretion of endorphin, a hormone that helps to feel psychological relief and excitement. Alan Lex, former director of the *Health Promotion Institute* in the United States, confirmed that helping others helps reduce the intensity of stress. Helping others reduces one's preoccupation with one's worries and problems and thus the person feels psychological comfort.

Now that we have learned that Islam cares about the social aspects, maintains the security of society, cohesion, and the spread of love, affection, sympathy, and compassion among believers, we have the opportunity to understand the importance of the words of the Almighty:

"And they give food in spite of love for it to the needy, the orphan, and the captive, [Saying], "We feed you only for the countenance of Allah. We wish not from you reward or gratitude!"(Qur'an, 76: 8-9)[208].

True maturity is after the age of forty

"And We have commended unto man kindness toward parents. His mother beareth him with reluctance and bringeth him forth with reluctance, and the bearing of him and the weaning of him is thirty months, till, when he

attaineth full strength and reacheth forty years, he saith: My Lord! Arouse me that I may give thanks for the favor wherewith Thou hast favored me and my parents and that I may do right acceptable unto Thee. And be gracious unto me in the matter of my seed. Lo! I have turned unto Thee repentant, and lo! I am of those who surrender (unto Thee). " (Qur'an 46:15) [209]

Psychological tests have shown that the total amount of deposited knowledge increases for the first 39 years of life, which reaches its peak at this time. So, before these psychological tests are done, Qur'an confirms that fact. It is interesting to know that the revelation to Muhammad ﷺ began in his forties and lasted for the next 23 years.

When considering this verse (divine verse) of the Qur'an, one should keep in mind the fact that the Qur'an was revealed at a time when all people had little scientific knowledge and no equipment to reach the correct description contained in the above verses.

After the age of forty, a person gradually begins to lose weight, just as he gradually became stronger. The Almighty said: *"Allah is He Who shaped you out of weakness, then appointed after weakness strength, then, after strength, appointed weakness and grey hair. He created what He will. He is the Knower, the Mighty."* (Qur'an, 30:45) [210]

Human strength lies between two weaknesses and life between two endings. First, the seed will be created, then it becomes an embryo, then a piece of meat, then a child in the mother's womb, and finally when it dies, it is called "sadig", or weak.

Circumcision as prevention

It is narrated from Abu Hurairah r.a. that the Prophet (peace and blessings of *Allaah be upon him*) said: *"Five things have been ordained by Allah for a man: circumcision, the removal of hair from the shy parts of the body, the cutting of the mustache, the cutting of the nails and the removal of the hair under the armpits."*[211]

It is known that Jesus himself was circumcised on the 8th day, as mentioned in the New Testament.

The United Nations has backed male circumcision as a way to prevent the spread of HIV among heterosexuals, saying the procedure should be made available to males in African countries. The World Health Organization and the United Nations AIDS Agency have backed recent research showing that removing the skin from the tip of the male genitalia can halve the risk of contracting HIV when having sex with infected women. They recommend that countries with a high rate of infected heterosexuals make this venture accessible to all who are interested, with younger, sexually active men preferred, but at the same time encouraging condom use and regular testing.

"These recommendations are a major step forward in HIV prevention," said Kevin De Cock, Director of the U.S. Centers for Disease Control and Prevention's (CDC) country mission in Kenya.[212] Out of the 40 million people living with HIV worldwide, 25 million live in Africa, where the virus is most commonly transmitted through sexual intercourse between heterosexual partners. The World Health Organization and the AIDS Agency say circumcision could stop the infection of 5.7 million men in the world over the next 20 years and save the lives of at least three million people. Worldwide, 30% of the male population is circumcised. Among Jews and Muslims, this procedure is performed for religious reasons, and in other communities for reasons of hygiene, and it is usually done in the first months of life.

The World Health Organization further points out that caution should be taken when explaining the protective effects of circumcision to people and that it should be made clear to both men and women that circumcision provides only partial protection.

The benefits of breast milk and breastfeeding

Mother milk is necessary for the first year.[213] Allah says: ***"And the mothers shall breastfeed their children (for) two years complete, for whoever wishes to complete the suckling... "*** (Qur'an 2:233)[214]
Good health and proper development of the baby depend on the quality and proper nutrition. Breast milk, which is ideal for the baby's nutritional needs, provides the necessary energy for its age, and also contains immune and components that protect it from diseases[215] and allergies. If the baby does not get enough milk or can not breastfeed at all, it should be supplemented or fed with adapted milk, for which it is necessary to consult a pediatrician. The worst food choice is plain cow's milk. Compared to breast milk, it differs significantly in the composition of proteins, fats, and carbohydrates and can cause serious problems. It is not recommended for the first year. Children with digestive problems are sensitive to cow's milk protein, which causes a variety of allergic reactions, so the only solution is food that does not contain cow's milk protein, such as soy protein-based milk.
In the second month, the baby slowly establishes its periodicity of meals, which is fewer than in the first month. In the third month, the baby has established a proper

breastfeeding cycle. From the fourth to the sixth month, the baby usually consume a larger amount of milk. After the fourth month, it can start drinking juices, porridge of vegetables, and fruits to slowly get used to other foods. It is a period when the baby needs to eat semi-solid food to learn to swallow and later to chew food. From 4 to 8 months, the baby should not eat salty foods so as not to damage the kidneys. During this period it should be given only natural fruit juices, which contain only natural sugar fructose. This avoids creating a desire for sugary foods. In babies with a tendency to allergies, the food that will be given additionally, should be hypoallergenic (with very little potential to cause an allergic reaction). Intense growth requires a change in diet. From the sixth to the eighth month, the baby's body is ready for beef and chicken porridge, which are an excellent source of protein and iron. Foods supplemented with dairy meals should be well mashed. From the age of eight months, the baby can start learning to drink from a cup. During this period, babies have their first teeth and the food they eat in addition to dairy meals does not have to be finely mashed.

Here we would also mention the ban on getting married between people who are related by milk. This applies to those who have been breastfed by the same mother. The harmfulness of such an act is confirmed in 1985 at the World International Congress. Once again the Superiority of the Qur'an is pointed out, and refers to the following quote:

- *"Prohibited to you [for marriage] are your mothers, your daughters, your sisters, your father's sisters, your mother's sisters, your brother's daughters, your sister's daughters, your [milk] mothers who nursed you, your sisters through nursing, your wives' mothers, and your step-daughters under your guardianship [born] of your wives unto whom you have gone in ... "* (Qur'an 4:23) [216]

Breast milk contains cells that carry genetic characteristics from both mother and father. This means that breast milk introduces traits from father and mother to the infant, which clarifies the Shari'a prohibition on marrying siblings because they had the same genetic traits even though they are not in any blood relationship. The research lasted a year and the team of experts who have investigated all of this was made up of seven medical doctors from the US and two from Egypt.

Marriage as a protection of human health

Marriage is a constant practice of Allah's Messenger ﷺ in which practical benefit is established for the spouses; they are kept away from fornication, building a family and offspring by continuing the human race and thus participating in the natural process that lasts until Judgment Day. There is no premarital, physical, intimate, sexual intercourse in Islam. It is strictly forbidden.

Allah, the Exalted, says: ***"And do not approach fornication."***[217] In an Islamic society that adhered to Islamic practice, adultery and prostitution were unknown. However, it should be emphasized that in Islam [218] there is also no asceticism, in the sense of ibadah[219] to give up sexual passions. They must be manifested and expressed only in a valid and legal marital union. The Messenger of Allah ﷺ rebuked the Companions who wanted to suppress their nature, in which Allah created them; with the need to eat, sleep, have intercourse with their wife's. When they said that they would give it up in favor of day and night worship, Prophet rebuked them and said to them: *"I worship and sleep, fast and eat, marry and do not give up*

from women, and who will abandon my sunnah[220] *and I give up from him. "*
The Prophet advised the Islamic youth with the following: *"Youth! Who can bear the marital obligations, let him get married, it is better to keep from the unlawful look and extramarital intercourse. He who cannot bear the burden and obligation of marriage, let him fast because it will be protection for him. "* Unfaithfulness and love affairs, which has become a kind of trend in the modern lifestyle, are great difficulties, and not only in terms of endangering marital idyll, but also increases the risk of heart disease. The increased risk is associated with stress, guilty conscience, evidence, and depression in those who cheat on their partners.

Although regular love life between spouses is very good for the heart, research from the University of Florence has found that it is not worth for married men and married women who cheat. Worse, their risk of heart attack is much higher because they face stressful and conflict situations.

Prohibited intercourse during the menstrual cycle

They ask you about menstruation: Say, it is harmful; you shall avoid sexual intercourse with the women during menstruation; do not approach them until they are rid of it. Once they are rid of it, you may have intercourse with them in the manner designed by God. God loves those who are clean. Your women are the bearers of your seed. Thus, you may enjoy this privilege however you like, so long as you maintain righteousness. You shall observe God, and know that you will meet Him. Give good news to the believers. [Qur'an 2:222-223] [221]

As we know, menstruation is a feminine issue. Ironically, it is the men who are mentioned and the revelation is directed towards the men. Now, what could concern a man regarding a feminine issue, except for his interest in sexual matters? God answers the men by initially letting them know that having sexual intercourse with a menstruating woman is harmful, and they should not approach them until they are clean.[12]

Medicine itself forbids doctors to perform examinations during a woman's menstrual cycle. A French women doctor noted that the inflammation of the reproductive organs in Christian women is far greater than in Jewish. She studied Christian and Jewish practices and noted that the reason for the increased disease among Christian women is because Jews do not approach their wives during the menstrual cycle,[222] while Christians do not pay attention to it. Menstrual discharge consists mainly of blood. It differs from ordinary blood in that it has more calcium and does not clot. It can also consist of microorganisms. Before leaving the body the content of menstruation was provided as food for the fetus. Menstruation is a positive symbol of a woman's ability to give birth to a child. But as it consists of not many ingredients that can support life, pathogenic microorganisms can also develop. Some ingredients, although not harmful, contain a very unpleasant odor. Intimate intercourse during menstruation is a huge risk. By changing some of the light secretions, some dangerous bacteria and viruses can be altered and as a result, diseases such as HIV and hepatitis can occur. They can be easily

---

[12]   Menstruation,   Sex,   Personal   Hygiene,   and   Quran
https://submission.org/Menstruation_2.html

transmitted if they come in contact with an open wound.[223]

The consequences of fornication on human health

Islam forbids fornication and prostitution and encourages marriage. The result of fornication is dangerous health consequences as well as the spread of immorality in society, and it is humiliation for women. Fornication is a feature of some animals and a perversion of some people, who, in addition to lying and betraying their spouse, can infect him with various diseases and their immoral life may cause their children and the generations after it to suffer from various diseases.

Allah says (interpretation of the meaning): ***"And do not approach fornication, for it is indecency, what a miserable path!"***[224]

Modern science has discovered many horrible diseases that cause fornication: syphilis, gonorrhea, itching. Syphilis leads to impotence, clogging of blood vessels, and angina pectoris. It is leading to hair loss and some times cause of abortion in women, and can lead to abnormalities or genetic atrophy in the fetus.

The tripper leads to sterility and inflammation of the genitals as well as rheumatism in young people, etc. Among the other diseases that have been studied are AIDS and the weakening of the immune system. This is all a result of prostitution, but also homosexuality.

It was narrated that 'Abdullah bin 'Umar said:

"The Messenger of Allah (ﷺ) turned to us and said: 'O Muhajirun, there are five things with which you will be tested, and I seek refuge with Allah lest you live to see them: Immorality never appears among a people to such an extent that they commit it openly, but plagues and diseases that were never known among the predecessors will spread among them. They do not cheat in weights and measures but they will be stricken with famine, severe calamity, and the oppression of their rulers. They do not withhold the Zakah of their wealth, but rain will be withheld from the sky and were it not for the animals, no rain would fall on them. They do not break their covenant with Allah and His Messenger, but Allah will enable their enemies to overpower them and take some of what is in their hands. Unless their leaders rule according to the Book of Allah and seek all good from that which Allah has revealed, Allah will cause them to fight one another.'"

AIDS is a terrible and horrifying disease and in Africa alone at least 6000 people die every day. The disease was discovered in the 80's of the last century and has spread across all continents. No effective cure or preventive vaccine has been found for this disease.

Ibn Abu Dunya narrates a narrationfrom the Messenger кот *"After shirk, there is no greater sin toward Allah than to leave one's seed in a womb that is not halal."*

Harm from homosexuality

Complete anomalies such as homosexuality, incest, etc. are mentioned in many places in the Qur'an, and their harmfulness and prohibition are extremely destructive to human nature and society in general. In those statements, the punishment that was reduced on that occasion is also mentioned.

That is related to the story of Lut a.s.[226] who was the grandson of Ibrahim a.s.[227] and was a believer and follower of Ibrahim as. When Ibrahim a.s. left his home in Chaldea and went to Syria and Palestine, Lut a.s. went with him into voluntary mission, running from persecution. The people of Lut a.s. who were obsessed with immorality laughed at him.

- *"...You have sex with men, .."*, and the answer of his *people was: "Make Allah's punishment to overtake us if you speak the truth!"* [228]

The Qur'an tells the story of how God destroyed the inhabitants of those cities except Lut ﷺ and the believers who followed him:

- *" Indeed, we will bring down on the people of this city punishment from the sky because they have been defiantly disobedient. And We have certainly left of it a sign as clear evidence for a people who use reason."* (Al Ankabut, 29: 34-35)

The punishment was sulfur rain, which completely covered their cities with possible earthquakes or volcanic eruptions. There is also a narration that says that the angel Gabriel a.s. raised that place with one wing to the sky and then flattened it. There is a place in the Bible called Sodom and Gomorrah. This destruction was to the point that the skeletons of humans found at the destroyed sites indicate fractures caused by strong pressure or impact from the air.

By disobeying God's rules, humanity, of which we are a part, faces the following diseases and illnesses, which by no means represent a healthy lifestyle! In America, it is estimated that 65 million people suffer from communicable diseases, which is about 21.3% of Americans, ie one-fifth of their population.

There are many types of sexually transmitted diseases and viruses that result from homosexuality. These include chlamydia, mycoplasma, ureaplasma, condyloma, genital herpes, urinary tract infections, scabies, lice, gonorrhea, syphilis, trichomoniasis, HIV, hepatitis B, hepatitis C, and etc.

This is just a confirmation of the words of the Messenger of Allah, may Allah bless him and grant him peace, who said: *"O group of Muhajireen, there are five things with which you will be tempted, and I ask Allaah to protect you from them: When fornication appears in a people and they spread to the extent that it is done publicly, a plague will appear in it, and diseases that did not exist among their ancestors who lived before!"*[229]

Nowadays, besides homosexual marriages,[230] there is adoption of children in cohabitation with homosexual couples. To meet their parenting needs, some government decide to let children raise in a homosexual environment. It has a great harmful effect on children and in psychology, this is called "modeling". What the children will see is considered correct and they will repeat the same pattern. It also contributes to the spread of this immoral and unnatural relationship that harms the normal development of the family and society.

Benefit from hijamah - cupping

A reciprocal treatment called Hijamah, or wet cupping, needs more tight guidelines and experienced experts. Hijamah is utilized to treat a wide scope of conditions including headaches and pain in the body, also treats blood pressure. It includes cutting the skin and drawing blood with pull cups.

The Messenger of God ﷺ reminded believers to treat themselves with hijamah:
" *"Indeed, hijamah is the best medicine you can use.."* At certain points, subcutaneous blood is pulled out, which regenerates rapidly in the body. He also said*: "If there is any good in your medicine, then it is in the incision with hijamah (pumping out blood) and a sip of honey." [Qur'an; Bukhari, 7/159.]."*[232]

is Cupping a practice that Muhammad ﷺ suggested to many people. Another narration that we can single out is the one when the Prophet ﷺ told the doctor Abu Ka'b to cut his skin and let bleed. Therefore the Prophet ﷺ said that: " *Hijamah(pulling out) cleanses the body from the outside while spilling blood cleanse the body from inside."* It should be performed when the stomach is empty and the person is fasting. It can be done due to headaches, migraines, and body aches, as well as during periods of mental strain. Normal blood flow improves human health. Otherwise, the human body continuously produces red blood cells and also, they increase, and the hijamah works to achieve balance in the blood, ie to expel unnecessary blood from the human body. The benefits of hijamah are as follows :

- Improving blood flow through the brain,
- Treating the blood cells,
- Stimulating the work of the liver, spleen and stomach,
- Treatment of muscle cramps in the neck, back, and legs,
- Treatment of migraine,
- By activating the blood circulation and improving its quality and increasing the immune system, the vision is improved and the eye diseases are treated,

- Treatment of general weakness,
- Treatment of diseases of the digestive system
- Treatment of nerve pain,
- Regulation of blood pressure,
- Freeing the body from bad blood,
- Activation of the immune system,
- Removal of toxins,
- Treatment of elevated uric acid,
- Treatment of damaged memory,
- Prevention of stroke.

Hijamah is a periodic process for cleansing the blood, which activates the cells and removes unnecessary toxins (poisons), and boosts the immune system.

The therapeutic effect of the Qur'an

The Islamic Organization of Medical Sciences in Kuwait has published the results of a scientific study that demonstrated to read the Qur'an to non-Muslims who do not understand the Arabic language has a therapeutic and calming effect. D-r.Ahmed Al Qhadij has presented the main results of his study at the special conference organized by the Islamic Community of North America.

He presented that physiological changes occurred in the neural system of patients who listened to the reading of the Qur'an while being controlled by an electronic modern system at a clinic in Panama, Florida.

He noted that the researcher conducted 120 experiments on five volunteers of both sexes, of different ages, who were not Muslims and did not speak Arabic. The experiment involved reading chapters from the Noble Qur'an in parallel with reading a plain Arabic text (which is not from the Qur'an). The volunteers did not know the difference between reading the Qur'an and reading the Arabic text. The Islamic medical doctor said that the experiments, which were performed by Dr. Al Qhadij have proved that 97% who listened to the reading of Qur'anic text had a stronger positive effect compared with subjects who only listened to plain Arabic text.

This shows the premise of any treatment is the Qur'an, as the essential methods, and afterward admittance to the next medication. It applies to a wide range of ailments, both mental and physical. Some accept that individuals whose ailment is physical ought to go to the clinic for treatment, while the individuals who are mentally sick should look for help in mental centers, and just for the mentally sick should the cure be in the Qur'an. On what premise did they make this division?

The Qur'an is a cure for sick hearts as well as for the vitality of human bodies. Allah, the Exalted, tells us: ***"We reveal in the Qur'an what is a cure and a mercy for the believers, and it only increases the calamity for the disbelievers."***[233]

They asked the Prophet Muhammad ﷺ about the Ruqyah(Qur'an therapy): " *O Messenger of God, the Ruqyah[234] which we use, the medicine we take, and the prevention we seek, does all this change Allah's precondition? He said, "They are part of Allah's planning."* [235] Let us look at the word " *schifaun* ", which is used here because of its visible result. And the word "*devaun*" (medicine) is not used, because for every medicine there is a possibility to use it sometimes, and sometimes not.

Ibn al-Qayyim in his book "*Zadul-ma'ad*" said: "In the Qur'an, there is a complete cure for all kinds of diseases, mental and physical. It is a cure for this world and hereafter. However, not everyone is praising Allah. If the patient wants to make proper use of the Qur'an for healing, he should impose it on his illness with firm faith and faith, sincerely and with complete confidence. Fulfilling these conditions, his illness will not be able to endure.

How can he oppose the word of the Lord of the heavens and the earth? How could he resist the war that would destroy the mountains if revealed to him, and cut the earth into pieces? Whomever the Qur'an does not cure, Allah does not cure, and to whom the Qur'an will not suffice, Allah will not make it on hand to him.[236]

This would mean that a good opinion of Allah and unlimited trust in Him is more than necessary during healing. *"The condition for the successful treatment of the patient is his firm belief that medicine will benefit him."*[237]

The lack of faith is seen in putting God's speech to the test, whether it will benefit us or not. If they drunk water from the ground out of pure taste and curiosity, it would not work. The complete certainty, conviction, and belief in our Lord will make the water healing for us.

Qur'anic recepie for healthy eating

Dr. Jamil Qudsi Duwyk[238] is a Palestinian nutritionist, claiming that the Qur'an answers every question, has written a more extensive 7,000-page Encyclopedia of *Islam* entitled *The Islamic Concept of Energy and Nutrition.*

Dr. Duwayk starts from the Qur'anic verses[239] , :

"We declare in the Qur'an what is a cure and a mercy for the believers, and it only increases the misfortune for the disbelievers."[240]

"Who created me and guided me to the right path, and who fed me and watered me, and who, when I am ill, heals me."[241]

Allah determined the word Moon to be mentioned 12 times in the Qur'an, exactly as many times as the number of months in a year. The word "day" is mentioned 365 times in the Qur'an, the word "prayers" (in the plural) five times as many as there are prayers in the day, the word "azm" (determination) five times, exactly as many times as the specially selected messengers of who have been given azm. Indeed, there are many such examples in the Qur'an. Dr. Duwayk says: "*Then, I said to myself, Allah (SWT), has a measure, which has been determined, then I will surely find the measure (formula) for food and drink from the Qur'an.*" He singled out all the verses that speak of eating and drinking. He concluded that the term eating is mentioned 109 times in the Qur'an, of which he singled out the haram foods mentioned 19 times, and obtained the number 90. He then listed all the types of food mentioned in the Qur'an, and how many types of food is mentioned and after a long analysis came to a fantastic discovery.

The number 90 represents the number of bites that each of us should take into the body every day for the body to function normally. In these 90 bites, there should be of all the types of food mentioned in the Qur'an, each type of food in such a large number of bites - how many times it is mentioned. For example, meat is mentioned 4 times, one bite weighs 20 to 25 grams, which means that you should eat 100 grams every day, no less, no more. Then the other types of food, exactly as much as specified in this Qur'anic recipe. Then he made a big table, which he divided into 240 squares, why the Qur'an is divided into 30 parts, each part into two parties, each party into 4 quarters, and he copied all the verses about one type of food into one square in which the first type of food, first mentioned. So he got 6 meals with an accurate list of foods, which would mean, ideally for each of us to eat 6 times a day - with smaller meals. Through that scheme, he came up with precise data on what to eat in the morning, what at noon, and what in the evening.

Lighter food is provided in the morning and stronger at midday, such as beans and meat, and in the evening only three things: dates, grapes, and pomegranate. According to Duwayk, there are general rules in the Qur'an that we should adhere to in our diet, ie food is always mentioned first and then after it, the drink, which means that the meal should start first with the food and end with the drink. Also, the fruit is always mentioned first and then after food, which means that a meal should always start with fruit and then with food.[242]

It is very interesting that in the Qur'an the meat of marine animals is always mentioned, before the meat of terrestrial animals. Dr. Duwayk in his extensive encyclopedia, explains many more rules, of which we emphasize the following:

-After milk, it is good to drink vinegar,

-Honey to be taken after the vinegar,

-Always eat dates after grapes, not the other way around, Pomegranate should always be the last thing we eat,

-Sour milk is better than sweet,

-Honey and milk should not be eaten together.

The mentioned project has also shown that in addition to strengthening the body's immunity, it also improves patient behavior.[243] Their mental state normalized very quickly. Among other things, tobacco addicts in just 21 days of treatment, very easily become non-smokers, because, their body simply refuses to receive everything unnatural and harmful.

Dr. Duvayk, among other things, teaches us how to make natural vinegar, skimmed sour milk, how to use wheat grain with husk, and the like.

Most importantly, the example of Dr. Duwayk educate us how to behave towards the Qur'an and how to study it. He called on Muslims, experts in various fields, to study the Qur'an from their profession and to discover the Qur'anic formula as the best solution for each field.

Mental illness

If we start mentioning the Qur'an as a remedy for diseases of the organs, our speech will be greatly lengthened. But we will mention some examples. There are some different diseases (mental and physical), to which Satan has a large share, due to his arbitrary and dictatorial behavior in our bloodstream. The Messenger of Allah said: *"Indeed, Shaytaan passes through the sons of Adam by circulating blood through the veins of men, so keep the Shaytaan hungry (fasting)."*[244]

The Prophet forbade superstition, pessimism, malice, talismans, divination, prophecy, looking at the stars and destiny, and magic. He said: *"Who will hang an amulet around his neck when he writes the companion of Allah; magic, talismans, and inscriptions are considered shirk."*[259]

The sorcery before the appearance of Muhammad ﷺ was widespread among the Arabs, but this type of expertise was completely rejected. A hadith states: "The *one who prophesies is a magician, the sorcerer is a fortuneteller, and the sorcerer is an unbeliever."*

Mental illness is the excitement of emotions, which, if they get too excited, become a precursor to Satan's touch, because it does not attack, except in irritated and excited nerves. Therefore, it is forbidden for a person to sleep alone and travel alone. It is mentioned in the hadith: *"One passenger is one devil, two passengers - two devils, only three passengers - are passengers."*

Dissociative identity disorder (DID)is a serious mental disorder that doctors try to cure with various pills and injections. To heal this kind of patient is difficult but possible. Suspicion is one of the many diseases most likely caused by the Jinn (which aims to break the human devotion to God). It begins with doubts about the correctness of ablution, prayer and ends with various doubts about belief. Treatment of doubts is with frequent mention of Allah (dhikr) and seeking refuge with Allah's name from Satan whispering with the words *"e'uzu billahi cross-devil-p-raid"* than to spit on the left side. Doing some useful things, maintaining family ties, as well as going out in the company of dear friends, will help a lot in avoiding the doubts that follow.

As for the real doubts (sensitive), they are much harder than imagined, because they cause pain in different parts of the patient's body. They are known among psychologists as "overwhelming" doubts. To cure them, it is necessary to add some specific things in the already mentioned ways.

For example, washing with cold water improves blood flow, exercise, sports, travel, movement, and anything that would in any way help to remove laziness, as well as creating an optimistic spirit through a gentle smile with your interlocutors and personal contentment with the provision of Allah. A person who fights against his doubts is like a warrior in the way of God. [260]

 God ordered us to do a specific deed: ***"Strike the ground with your foot - and here is cold water for bathing and drinking!"***[261]

To remove our doubts, there is no obstacle to using certain remedies, if we are simply forced to do so. But it is important to note that it brings only a one-time calming, not the final cure. They are included in the Shari'ah permitted means of health treatment, which we combine with the basic method of treatment.

The cure for depression is often found in mosques. The Prophet (peace and blessings of Allah be upon him) said: *"The joy of my heart is in prayer."*[262] The jinns are always trying to pull the man into solitude so that they can control him more easily. That is why Islam forbade people to spend the night alone, to travel alone, and so on. When the devils fail to control a person, they drag him into subconscious loneliness, and, the person feels lonely, even in the presence of other people. As a result, such people become more and more distracted, and their thoughts become disordered.[263]

From this, we conclude that anger is the cause of many diseases. For this reason, a man came to the Prophet asking him to advise him on something useful, and he said to him: *"Do not get angry!"* This sentence he repeated several times.[245] The scars that anger leaves on a personal history are always visible.

Likewise, incredible annoyance brings a sort of colon spasm, while diabetes in certain individuals is activated by incessant extreme excitement. Numerous ailments of the head, for example, migraine, stroke, dribble, and abrupt loss of motion, are ailments brought about by outrage. Here we will include a couple of more heart maladies, for example, angina and angina pectoris. Outrage assumes a significant part in making these illnesses just as their irritation. In a word, it is the reason for all irregularities, since it originates from Satan.

Allah, the Exalted, said: ***"And remember Our servant Job when he cried to his Lord: 'Satan indeed touches me with sorrow and suffering."***[246] Ayub or Job, peace be upon him, is said to have been afflicted with all sorts of mental and physical ailments. The words "with sorrow and suffering" (*bi nusubin ve azabin) is* to mean painful and exhausting, with mental suffering due to illness. He attributed all this to Satan because he is the cause of his severe temptation.[247]

The teaching of the Qur'an has been implemented over many sick people who have suffered from various diseases, especially those who are called incurable, and for whom there is a great belief that they were caused by Satan. Some of these diseases are: cancer, the consequences of a heart

145

attack, chronic asthma, paralysis, infertility, diabetes and all have been cured by the grace of God.

Irregular menstruation in some women, whether it is delayed or prolonged, for no particular reason, is usually caused by a jinn[248] . The Prophet (peace and blessings of Allaah be upon him) was asked about it. He told Hamni bint Jahsh, when she complained of unusually heavy bleeding during menstruation: *"It is a sting of Satan stings."*[250] Satan attempts to prolong the duration of the bleeding by partially delaying menstruation and to prevent the woman from worshiping and studying the Qur'an. Another way it is used is to injure a part of a vein. In this case, the woman is confused and fails to distinguish between menstrual blood and plain blood and consequently stops praying. Similar to this case is the example of paralysis. The Jinn presses a part of the patient's body so that he is no longer able to move it.

Also, there are frequent side effects such as major depression, anxiety, and subsequent headaches. If one was to study the Qur'an, such a patient would feel chills in his paralyzed body. In case they did not feel any reaction, it would mean that the Jinn left his body, but previously damaged nerve fibers, due to which the body remained like that (paralyzed). Such difficult and complicated situations require a lot of patience and unceasing learning of the Qur'an, with a sincere intention of healing.

Each of these verses can be recited, just as any other verse from the Qur'an which can help heal these diseases. Proof of this are the words of the Messenger of Allah, addressed to Aisha, when a woman came to her for medicine: *"Treat her with the help of the Book of Allah."*[258]

Conclusion

All that is stated is not to propagate and call for the abandonment of the usual way of treatment, such as going to the hospital for diagnosis and medical treatment. On the contrary. In this book, you were briefly introduced to the alternative and natural ways of healing that come from a divine choice and God's pharmacy full of wisdom. We have all witnessed reading this work with the subtlety of modern knowledge and recommendations given to us by the Last Messenger of God with his wise advice. Surgically, we have pointed out the paths and the direction we need to follow to reach our happiness. That happiness is not possible without physical and spiritual health. We have seen that the basis of all healing is trough God's revelation and what is mentioned in the traditional ways of healing. We are convinced that hygiene and health can not be without each other, just as spirituality can not be separated from morality.

Modern medicine and natural treatments are today a sublimation that has evolved into a new kind of alternative medicine. Nowadays, more than ever, we have the task of acquainting people with the benefits of Islamic medicine when many people have lost faith in finding the cure they are looking for. Sometimes the medicine is within our reach and is completely free. It only takes a little time. It is necessary to step a little beyond our vanity and understanding of the world that doctors, hospitals, health institutions are not the only ones responsible for our health. It is primarily our duty in this global world of change, technological advantages, but also challenges. We owe it to ourselves to protect our health, our families, and our friends, and information is a tool that can help us overcome many difficulties. Islamic civilization and the Prophet's timeless seed of advice's are a good starting point for understanding a new concept of healing that has worked for hundreds of years and helped man overcome numerous consequences.

Note

[1] One of the most beautiful things that Islam prescribes is that after the mention of any Messenger of Allah, a short prayer should be said: " ﷺ " (sallallaahu 'alayhi wa sallam). This means: "May Allah's blessings and peace be upon him."
[2] One of the scholars who followed the Hanbali school of law in Islam. Especially prominent for its knowledge of the traditions dating back to the time of Muhammad ﷺ.
[3] Reported by Imam Ahmed in his Musnad. Reported by Ahmad and the six sunnah. Tirmidhi considers it a sound hadith.
[4] It is narrated in an Israelite (a tradition passed down from the followers of the Book) that the close friend of God Ibrahim (Abraham), peace be upon him, asked Allah Almighty: "My Lord, where does the disease come from?" And Allah replied: " from me! "Ibrahim asked again:" How did the remedy come? "God replied:" also from me", what about the doctor? "asked Ibrahim then Allah replied," It is through man u which I send medicine. "
[5] Transmitted by Muslim.
[6] Allah - God, the supreme and only God, Lord and Creator, known in Christianity as the Father, and in Judaism as Yahweh.
[7] Reported by Muslim in his Sahih.
[8] El Ijaz et Tibbi.
[9] Muslim scholars have written a lexicon-like work or encyclopedia with a dictionary of the names of various plants, in Arabic, Greek, Syrian, Persian, and Berber, and a dictionary explaining the names of natural remedies, ie medicines that are not composed of various artificial components. To the medicines known before, they added some medicines that they invented and wrote the first books on

medicinal herbs. (Xhelal Muzhir, Hadaratul - Islami ve eseruha fit - tere kkil - ilm, p.306)

[10] Lubon Gustav, The *Civilization of the Arabs,* p. 494.

[11] Xhelal Muzhir, Hadaratul *Islami ve eseruha fit terekkil ilmi* , p. 312.

[12] The word "muhtesib" (inspector) in its original Arabic form is still used in Spain today.

[13] In his book Natural Remedies, he collected and studied various plants and medicines from the Mediterranean coast, Spain, and Syria. In his book, he noted one thousand four hundred medicinal plants and compared the findings with one hundred and fifty Arab scholars. It was the result of an in-depth study and precise observation with extensive scientific knowledge.

[14] Mebhasut - tibb, menshurun fit-turasil - islamiyji bi israfi, Arnold, p.485

[15] Some of those ways are: Distillation with crystallization.

[16] Ferdi Tufan *Ulemaul ara bi ve ma eatavhu lil-hadara,* p. 27-28.

[17] Dr. Ragib es – Serdjani.

[18] In the work *Compendium on Remedies* Ibn al-Baytar spoke about the use of the drug, it's a beneficial but also harmful effect, pointing to various types of plants from which various essential oils are obtained by processing, such as rose, wormwood an etc.

[19] In this review of the plant world, he has at hand the work of Greek and Arab botanists: Dioscorides, Galen, Hunayn ibn Ishaq, Ibn Shizaun, Ibn Juljul, Az-Zahrawi, and others.

[20] In addition to this work, Ibn Sina wrote many other works, including: " *The Book of Healing* ", " *Remedies for Cardiovascular Diseases* ", " *The Work of Intestinal Diseases* ", etc.

[21] Wikipedia.

[22] Reported by Ahmed in his Musnad.

[23] Reported by Ahmad ibn Abdullah ibn Umar r.a.

[24] This world, earthly life.

[25] Afterlife, life after death.

[26] The narration is narrated from Abu Fadil al-Abbas ibn Abdulmuttalib, r.a.

[27] Reported by Bukhari.

[28] i.e. followers.

[29] Ahmed in his Musnad, Hakim in his Mustederek.

[30] Sovereign.

[31] Listen to what Allah's Messenger says: *"Healthy people on Judgment Day would wish their bodies were cut with scissors and pliers when they see the reward of those who were tempted on the Earth)."* (Tirmidhi, Sahih).

[32] Reported by Muslim.
[33] The practical act of prayer.
[34] Ritual washing of the body with water.
[35] Bukhari and Muslim.
[36] Bukhari and Muslim.
[37] Bukhari, Muslim and Nesai.
[38] Ibn Majah and Hakim (saheeh)
[39] Qur'an; 41/53 .
[40] Pain which is especially great is also described in the Qur'an as a punishment for those who will end up in the Fire of Hell:" *..we will replace them with other skins, to feel the real punishment! And Allah is the Mighty, the Wise." (Qur'an 4/56)*
[41] The hadith is narrated by al-Tirmidhi.
[42] Tirmidhi, Abu Dawud.
[43] Thyme.
[44] In addition to Antimony, Turkish scientists have found that flaxseed protects the eyes. Flaxseed contains ten nutrients, including omega-3 and omega-6 fatty acids, vitamins B1, B2 and C, iron and zinc.

[45] Qur'an; El Wakia, 29.
[46] Qur'an, Kaf, 10.
[47] Qur'an, Rahman, 68.
[48] Companions - the first generation of Muslims who saw

Muhammad ﷺ directly, accompanied him, learned from him,

followed him most correctly, and most consistently in his actions (Ref.).
[49] Reported by Bukhari.
[50] Qur'an, An-Nahl, 10-11.
[51] Qur'an, An-Nahl,
[52] Ibn Majah.
[53] Ibn Majah.
[54] Ibn Majah.
[55] Quran, One entails E exp, 17.
[56] i.e. heaven.
[57] Qur'an, Al Insan, 17-18.
[58] Qur'an, 36/ 33.
[59] Qur'an, 50/9.
[60] Qur'an; Rahman, 12-13.
[61] Bukhari.
[62] Reported by Aisha r.a.
[63] Qur'an; El Enam, 99.
[64] Transmit Abu Nuaim through Anas RA.
[65] Abdurahman Es Sujuti, *Vjerovesnikova medicina* , Libris, Sarajevo, 2003, p.76

[66] Translated by Aliy r.a. and Nuaim.

[67] Iron needs vary at different times in life. Most iron is needed during the growing period, ie. children and teenagers need the most iron. Also, pregnant women and women with heavy menstruation should get more iron.

Allaah says **(interpretation of the meaning)**: *"And We created the iron, in which it has great power, and it is for the benefit of mankind - and that Allah may guide those who* believe in *Him and His messengers when they do not see Him"* (Qur'an, 57/25)

[68] Et Tirmidhi and Beyheki.

[69] Abu Dawud.

[70] Bukhari, 495.

[71] Tirmidhi narrates the hadith through Ausha r.a. A similar hadith is narrated through Enes r.a.

[72] Qur'an, Tin (Fig), 1-2.

[73] Indicates that it grows without human care or cultivation.

[74] Reported by al- Bukhaari and Muslim.

[75] Among other things, there is a kind of legend that truffles can not be grown, that is, that the seeds thought to be from truffles do not yield any harvest. There is also another story that in 1808 truffles were successfully cultivated in France, by growing a certain type of tree in which truffle roots were found.

[76] The specimens you can see in the Mycology Laboratory in Skopje do not look impressive at all: the mushrooms are small, ugly and do not smell very pleasant (roughly, of garlic and old cheese).

[77] Muslim.

[78] Muslim.

[79] Scientific experiments have shown that dates contain stimulants that strengthen the muscles of the uterus in the last months of pregnancy. This helps the uterus to expand at the time of delivery on the one hand and to reduce postpartum hemorrhage on the other. Dates stimulate the uterus by regulating it and speed up labor contractions. The uterus is a relatively large muscular organ and urgently requires an adequate supply of natural sugar during labor and delivery. As laxatives, dates are very important for a pregnant woman and before childbirth to cleanse the colon and help with childbirth. (note av.)

[80] Bukhari and Muslim narrate a hadith from Anas ibn Malik says: "A child was born, and Abu Talha told me, 'Take it to the Messenger ﷺ sending dates. "The Messenger of God took it, ate the dates, then took them out of his mouth and put them in the mouth of the child, rubbed his gums, and named him Abdullah."

[81] This is evidenced by the British Medical Journal, which on June 10, 1995, published a study by a group of English scientists conducted at a hospital in the city of Leeds.

[82] Abu Dawud.

[83] Reported by Abu Dawud.

[84] Virgin Mary, mother of Jesus, peace be upon her.

[85] Angel.

[86] Nigella Sativa, black seed, kalonji, ar: el-habetu es-sevda.

[87] Bukhari, 7/160. This hadith of the Prophet, Lj (narrated by Abu Hurairah, in a Saheeh narration, and recorded by Bukhari and Muslim) is credited with the immense popularity of black seed in the Islamic world, which is also called the blessed grain. Modern science today confirms the correctness of this hadith.

[88] The medical part of the *Canon medicinae* collection in the 11th century was of enormous importance for the establishment of medicine as a science and was considered the most important medical textbook in Europe for the next 500 years.

[89] The immunologist Dr. Peter Schleicher is the author of the book: "Black Cumin: A Magical Egyptian Plant for Allergies, Asthma, Skin Diseases, and Immune Problems."

[90] Ali BH, Blunden G (2003). Pharmacological and toxicological properties of *Nigella sativa. Phytother Res* , **17** , 299-305.

[91] El-Mahdy MA, Zhu Q, Wang QE, et al (2005). Thymoquinone induces apopt*osis through activation of caspase-8 and mitochondrial events in p53-null myeloblastic leukemia HL-60 cells. Int J Cancer, 117,* 409-17.

[92] Salim, EI, Fukushima, S (2003). Chemopreventive potential of volatile oil from black cumin (*Nigella sativa* L.) seeds against rat colon carcinogenesis. *Nutr Cancer*, **45**, 195-202.

[93] Salomi MJ, Nair SC, Panikkar KR (1991). Inhibitory effects of *Nigella sativa* and saffron (Crocus sativus) on chemical carcinogenesis in mice. *Nutr Cancer*, **16**, 67-7 2.

[94] Chehl N, Chipitsyna G, Gong Q, et al (2009). Anti-inflammatory effects of the *Nigella sativa* seed extract, thymoquinone, in pancreatic cancer cells. *HPB* , **11** , 373-81.

[95] Awad EM (2005). *In vitro* decreases of the fibrinolytic potential of a cultured human fibrosarcoma cell line, HT1080, by *Nigella sativa* oil. *Phytomedicine*, **12**, 100-7.

[96] Khan N, Sultana S (2005). Inhibition of two stages renal carcinogenesis, oxidative damage and hyperproliferative response by *Nigella sativa. Eur J Cancer Prev*, **14**, 159-68.

[97] Ahmad D, Abulkhair O, Nemenqani D, et al (2012). antiproliferative properties of methanolic extract of *Nigella sativa*

against the MDA-MB-231 cancer cell line. *Asian Pac J Cancer Prev*, **13**, 5839-42.

[98] Swamy SM, Huat BT (2003). Intracellular glutathione depletion and reactive oxygen species generation a re important in alpha-header in-induced apoptosis of P388 cells. *Mol Cell Biochem*, **245**, 127-39.

[99] Mabrouk GM, Moselhy SS, Zohny SF, et al (2002). Inhibition of methyl nitrosourea (MNU) induced oxidative stress and carcinogenesis by orally administered bee honey and Nigella grains in Sprague Dawley rats. *J Exp Clin Cancer Res*, **21**, 341-6.

[100] Al-Sheddi ES, Cytotoxicity of Nigella Sativa Seed Oil and Extract Against Human Lung Cancer Cell Line, DOI: http://dx.doi.org/10.7314/APJCP.2014.15.2.983

[101] Bukhari and Muslim.

[102]   Chest pain during inhalation.

[103] Qur'an, An Nakhl, 66.

[104] Koran 16 / 14.

[105] Transmit Ibn Babe.

[106] Reported by Abu Dawud.

[107] This will give you the same results as eating fish or lean white meat, in terms of lowering total and bad cholesterol (LDL), thereby reducing the risk of heart disease.

[108] Qur'an, Anne Nakhl, 68-69.

[109] Honey consists of sugar, glucose, and fructose, minerals such as magnesium, potassium, calcium, sodium chloride, sulfur, iron, and phosphates. It also contains vitamin B1, B2, C, B6, B5, and B3, and the concentration of all of the above depends on the quality of the nectar and pollen. Honey in small quantities also contains copper, iodine, and zinc. Therefore, it contains and several types of hormones.

[110] Bukhari and Muslim.

[111] Noted by Bukhari and Muslim by Abu Sa'id al-Khudri .

[112] The hadith was recorded by Ibn Majah and Hakim, the hadith is sahih - authentic.

[113] *Dr. Javier Menendez* from the Catalan Oncology Institute and *Dr. Antonio Segura Carretero* of the University of Granada, examining which ingredients are most effective against breast cancer, found that quality unrefined olive oil contains many "phytochemical" ingredients that can cause malignant cell death.

[114] Dlalelal uddin Abdurrahman es-Sujuti, *Vjerovjesnikova medicina* , Libris, Sarajevo, 2003., p. 71-72.

[115] Hadith narrated by Abu Nuaym.

[116] Ahmed, No. 16529.

[117] Qur'an, Al-Ma'ida, 6; Also: " **Allah truly loves those who repent often and loves those who are very clean.** (Al-Baqarah, 222)

[118] Abu Dawud, Ahmed, 'Abdulaziz, and At Tabarani. Reliable and well-known collections of legends. (note).

[119] Earth - the source located next to the Frog (note)

[120] Tirmidhi notes that it is a good narration.

[121] Qur'an 14:37.

[122] Notes Ahmed and Ibn Majah

[123] Japanese researcher and scientist Dr. Mesaru Imuti, who was the director and president of the Hadu Institute for Scientific Research in Tokyo, visited Saudi Arabia and gave a lecture at the Darul Hikme University, which was attended by more than 500 top scholars. and researchers also confirmed that he had performed several experiments on Earth-water (which he had obtained from some Arabs).

[124] In the name of Allah (SWT)

[125] kaheel7.com/eng/index.php/secrets-of-Qur'an-a -sunnah / 287- the-memory-of-zamzam-water

[126] Imam Bukhari cites an authentic tradition of Aisha and Maimun (r.a.), that the Prophet (a) while bathing (gushul) he first washed his hands, and in one tradition also the full organ, then he washed his mouth and throat and took ablution as ablution is taken for prayer. Afterward, he washed his head, and after that his whole body so that nothing was left dry.

[127] Ibn Majah and Ahmed.

[128] Practice of the Prophet

[129] Ritual washing with water

[130] i.e. The devil.

[131] Abdurezak 10/427 hadith; 19588.

[132] Muslim.

[133] Followers, people.

[134] Ahmed, Hassan.

[135]   Miswak is derived from the arak tree and is also the best species of miswak. It has a special smell and taste. This tree grows in warm tropical regions, in Saudi Arabia, Sudan, Pakistan, and East India.

[136] i.e. practice.

[137] Special wood used for brushing teeth.

[138] Before each prayer, at least 5 times a day.

[139] Reported by Beyheki.

[140] Reported by Muslim.

[141] Qur'an, Baqare, 172.

[142] Qur'an, Al-Baqarah, 173.

[143]   The antonym of this word is the word " haram " or forbidden.

[145] Part of the text was used by Dr. Monika Samardzioska, www.rak.mk.com

[146] Qur'an, Al-Baqarah, 173.

[147] Bible, Leviticus laws, 11: 7-8.

[148] Bible, Deuteronomy, 14: 8.

[149] Qur'an, As-Saff, 47.

[150] Allah, the Exalted, says: O believers, wine, dice, idols, and divination arrows are abominations, the work of Satan; so avoid them to achieve what you want. Satan wants to bring enmity and hatred between you with the help of wine and wine and to divert you from the remembrance of Allah and from performing the prayer. Well, will you stop? (El Maida, 91-92)

[151] Narrated Tabarani by Abdullah ibn Amr.

[152] Ahmed records a narration from Umar ibn al-Khattab.

[153] Nasai in his Sunan.

[154] Gabriel - the angel Gabriel, who was commissioned by God to deliver revelations to God's Messengers and Believers.

[155] Ahmed, Hakim, and Bayhaq and quoted by Ibn Abbas.

[156] Recorded by Muslim, Abu David, and Tirmidhi.

[157] Proverbs 20: 1.

[158] Ephesians 5:18.

[159] The research is based on data from the Fatality Analysis Reporting System (FARS). The data includes information on 1,495,667 people who were in a serious car accident between 1994 and 2008. What is interesting is that the FARS covers the entire American nation, every day of the week, all parts of the day, and the report of the quantities for alcohol in the "units of measurement" of 0.01% in the blood. (note)

[160] Consuming just 1.25 decilitres of wine a day increases the risk of cancer by a staggering 168%! This is the conclusion reached by French oncologists, and more detailed results are published in the report of the National Cancer Institute (INCA).

[161] Ibn Majah, no.3362.

[162] Legal act

[163] Buhari 5157 and Muslim, 3727.

[164] The study was conducted on men between the ages of 18 and 44 and is the first such study in the world. The study included 369 testicular cancer patients who were surveyed for cannabis consumption. The results were compared with 979 healthy men who did not have testicular cancer. The study found that cannabis was linked to testicular cancer, regardless of cigarette smoking, alcohol consumption, and a positive family history of the disease (heredity). Researchers at the British Cancer Research Center said the study was the first to link testicular cancer to cannabis and involved a small number of respondents.

[165] Tirmidhi, Ibn Majah

[166] The Prophet's Medicine - Ibn Qayyim Al-Jawzi

[167] Reported by Abu Dawud.

[168] Pre- Islamic Arabs often practiced divination when traveling on the road, in trade, when seeking to marry or engage in any important business, or with special arrows located in the Kaaba with priests. The Qur'an forbids all divination and prediction of the future.

[169] Qur'an, El Maida, 3.

[170] www.nhs.uk

[171] "The Basic Values of Ramadan Fast."

[172] Qur'an, Al-Najm, 59-60.

[173] Qur'an, Al-Mutafifin, 6.

[174] i.e. Throne.

[175] This research was published in the International Journal of Psychiatry in Medicine, which is an important scientific source in the field of medicine, and concluded that people who describe themselves as infidels get sick much faster and their life expectancy is very short.

[176] Herbert Benson and Mark Stark, Timeless Healing (New York: Simon & Schuster, 1996), 203.

[177] Qur'an, 13 / 28.

[178] Qur'an; El Ahzab, 44.

[179] Glynn, Patrick. *God: The Evidence: The Reconciliation of Faith and Reason in a Postsecular World.* 1999.

[180] Ibn Qayyim, *Treasury of Knowledge.*

[181] Muttefequn alayhi.

[182] Qur'an, 2 / 155-156 .

[183] Q renesuva Abu Hurejre .

[184] Acts of Worship of Almighty God.

[185] Sahih al-Jami'a, 4079

[186] Narration of Tabarani (Albani rated as credible)

[187] Kazim, Ebrahim. *The modern-day problem of electromagnetic waves: Prostration on the ground the solution?* https://eliehouse.wordpress.com/2010/12/17/modern-day-problem-of-electromagnetic-waves-prostration-on-the-ground-the-solution.

[188] By placing the head of the country with falling prostrate on his forehead and nose.

[189] http://www.nur-islam.com/

[190] Transmitted ute Ahmed Ibn Sa'di.

[191] Qur'an, Er-Rahman, 76.

[192] Diab, DA (2015, dec 15) .www.Qur'an-m.com. Retrieved from www.Qur'an-m.com: http://www.Qur'an-m.com.

[193] www.55a.net

[194] Qur'an, 74/7.

[195] And Allah will protect them from the fear of that Day, and will grant them bliss and joy (76/11)

[196] Tirmidhi, no.1879.

[197] Tirmidhi

[198] Qur'an; Ali Imran, 134.

[199] Qur'an; Heaven, 9.

[200] Qur'an; Furkan, 47.

[201] Qur'an; Rum, 23.

[202] Reported by El Bezar.

[203] Tirmidhi.

[204] Reported by al -Tabarani .

[205] Transmit Abu Dawud, An-ute Ibn Huzejme and others.

[206] Bukhari, no.12 and Muslim, no.64.

[207] Bukhari, no.5559 and Muslim, no.67.

[208] Qur'an; Ed-Dehr, 8-9.

[209] Qur'an, 46/15.

[210] Qur'an, Rum, 54.

[211] Bukhari and Muslim.

[212] http://www.wipo.int

[213] Breastfeeding helps with pain in infants. Researchers in Mount Sinai, Toronto, believe that breastfeeding helps relieve pain in newborns. Namely, the research was conducted on over 1000 babies over whom a blood sample was taken with a needle, after which it was shown how breastfeeding affects relieving pain. Heart rate and respiration rate as well as the duration of crying after needle stabbing were examined. It is possible that the calming is influenced by the taste of milk, as well as the secretion of endorphins, a chemical that is a natural painkiller (www.plivazdravje.hr)

[214] Qur'an, Al-Baqarah, 233.

[215] Breastfeeding reduces the risk of heart disease. This was done by British scientists from the Child Health Institute, which involved more than 200 teenagers. The same goes for some other diseases such as respiratory diseases, stroke, high blood pressure, diabetes, etc. (www.vasezdravlje.com)

[216] Qur'an; Ann Nisa, 23.

[217] Qur'an; Al-Isra, 32.

[218] Islam - the name of the only religion recognized by God. Islam means submission, tranquility, and peace .

[219] Ibadah - worship, slavery, total obedience, and devotion to the Creator. In this case, we mean the God-pleasing deeds, deeds of great piety with which God is pleased (Ref.).

[220] Sunnah - the tradition of God's Messenger Muhammad ﷺ.

[221] Qur'an; El Bekare, 222.

[222] But of course they exaggerate and treat them like animals, neither eating nor drinking with them, but completely isolating them.

[223] www.medicina.hr

[224] Qur'an; El Isra, 32 .

[225] Ibn Majah, Bezar and Bayhaqi record a narration from Ibn 'Umar, *Et tergibu wa Terhib* , p.109

[226] Lot.

[227] Abraham.

[228] Qur'an; El Ankebut, 29.

[229] Transmit Ibn Madjah.

[230] Statistically, the number of gay marriages in the United States is increasing today:
646,000 - Number of gay households in the United States in 2010, according to the Household Census Bureau - Source: CNN
80.4% - Growth in the percentage of gay households in the United States between 2000 and 2010, according to the Household Census Bureau - Source: CNN
115,064 Number of gay households with children in the United States, according to the Household Census Bureau: CNN.

[231] Muslim

[232] Qur'an; Bukhari, 7/159.

[233] Qur'an, Al-Isra, 82.

[234] Islamic prayer formula used for healing.

[235] I have Ahmed in his Musnad and Sunan on Tirmidhi.

[236] Ibn Qayyim al-Jawziyyah - Zadul-ma'ad, 4/352

[237] Zadul-me'ad, 4/98

[238] Dr. Jamil Qudsi Dweik

[239] Verse - quote or verse from the Qur'an. So a sign or proof .

[240] Qur'an; Al-Isra, 82.

[241] Qur'an; Ash-Shuara, 78-80.

[242] *"and with his help gardens of palms and vines for you elevate - they have a lot of fruits and you eat -"* (Al Muminun, 23/19)
The fruit also protects against radiation. This was determined by NASA researchers working to increase the protection of spacecraft from radiation. Their experiments with experimental mice showed that mice fed strawberries, blueberries, kale, and spinach were less prone to neurological damage than other mice.

[243] It is important to note that Dr. Duveijk has practically confirmed his theory of healing and preserving health by using the Qur'anic recipe for nutrition. He offered the mentioned way to 200 sick people who were suffering from incurable diseases of both physical and mental nature. After only 21 days he got amazing results. The percentage of completely cured was 90%, and the other patients felt a great

improvement. Among the patients were those with diabetes, rheumatisms, those who had problems with their joints, lungs, or had cancer, and so on.

[244] Reported by Ahmad (Muttefeku n alayhi).

[245] The hadith was recorded by Bukhari

[246] Qur'an; Saad, 41.

[247] Al-mu'jamu al-mufahrezu li al-fazi al-Qur'an al-Karim, Hasan Ali Karimah, p. 132

[248] Gene - spiritual being invisible, daemon (note. On av.).

[249] Reported by Abu Dawud.

[250] Transmits Tirmidhi.

[251] Sahih Muslim, 14/189.

[252] Qur'an; Hood, 44.

[253] "Zadul-mead" 4/358.

[254] Qur'an; Esh-Shu'ara, 80.

[255] Qur'an; El-Inshikak, 3-5.

[256] Qur'an; Al-Inshirah, 1-3.

[257] Qur'an; Ez-Zilzal, 1.

[258] "E s-silsiletu es-sahihatu", El-Albani, 1931.

[259] Believing in something equal to Allah is the work of paganism.

[260] Qur'an; Saad, 41.

[261] Qur'an; Saad, 42.

[262]   Musnad of Imam Ahmed, 5/364

[263] As our speech on the treatment of all kinds of diseases with the help of the Qur'an would not be delayed, I suggest that anyone who wants to know more about it should refer to the work "Zadul-me'ad", the fourth book (Kitabut- tib), from Ibn al-Qayyim. (Note av.)